MINIMAL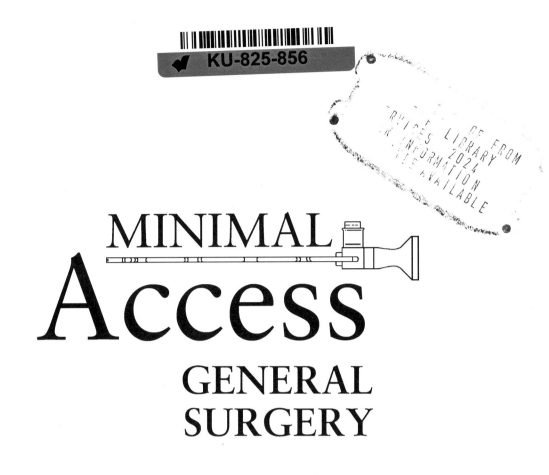
Access
GENERAL
SURGERY

Edited by R David Rosin MS, FRCS, FRCS(Ed)
St Mary's Hospital, London

Foreword by Frederick Greene

RADCLIFFE MEDICAL PRESS, OXFORD AND NEW YORK

© 1994 Radcliffe Medical Press Ltd
15 Kings Meadow, Ferry Hinksey Road, Oxford OX2 ODP

Radcliffe Medical Press, Inc
141 Fifth Avenue, New York, NY 10010, USA

British Library Cataloguing in Publication Data

A cataloguing record for this book is available from the British Library.

ISBN 1 870905 72 5

Library of Congress Cataloging in Publication Data

Minimal access general surgery/edited by R David Rosin; foreword by Frederick Greene.
    p. cm.
  Includes bibliographic references and index.
  ISBN 1 870905 72 5 (cased): $90.00
  1. Endoscopic surgery.   I. Rosin, R. David.
  [DNLM: 1. Surgery, Operative - methods. ". Surgery, Laparoscopic - methods. WO 500
    M6642 1994]
  RD33.53.M55 1994
  617'.05-dc20
  DNLM/DLC   93-41152

Typeset by Bookman, Slough
Printed and bound in Great Britain by
Biddles Ltd, Guildford and King's Lynn

Dedicated to

My late father, Mr IR Rosin OBE, MD, FRCS (Ed),

an inspiration, guide and true renaissance surgeon

Contents

List of Authors

Maurice E Arregui, St Vincent Hospital, Indianapolis, Indiana, USA

Huba Bajusz, The General Infirmary, Leeds, UK

R Belliard, Centre de Chirurgie Laparoscopique, Bordeaux, France

Sarah Cheslyn-Curtis, Luton and Dunstable Hospital, London, UK

D Collet, Centre de Chirurgie Laparoscopique, Bordeaux, France

Bernard Dallemagne, Clinique Saint Joseph, Liège, Belgium

J Desplantez, Centre de Chirurgie Laparoscopique, Bordeaux, France

M Edye, Centre de Chirurgie Laparoscopique, Bordeaux, France

David R Fletcher, Austin Hospital, Melbourne, Australia

M Mounir Gazayerli, Laparoscopic Laser Surge-on Institute, Troy, Michigan, USA

Mohamed Hakki, Egypt Air Hospital, Cairo, Egypt

Hosam S Helmy, Cairo University, Cairo, Egypt

Namir Katkhouda, University of Southern California School of Medicine, Los Angeles, California, USA

Patrick F Leahy, Blackrock Clinic, Dublin, Eire

E Magne, Centre de Chirurgie Laparoscopique, Bordeaux, France

Michael J McMahon, The General Infirmary, Leeds, UK

Jean Mouiel, Hospital Saint-Roch, Nice, France

Jorge L Navarrete, St Vincent Hospital, Indianapolis, Indiana, USA

J Perissat, Centre de Chirurgie Laparoscopique, Bordeaux, France

Joseph B Petelin, Surgix, Shawnee Mission, Kansas, USA

Lothar W Popp, Clinic Dr Guth, Hamburg, Germany

John A Rennie, King's College Hospital, London, UK

David Rosin, St Mary's Hospital, London, UK

Christopher Russell, The Middlesex Hospital, London, UK

Humphrey J Scott, St Mary's Hospital, London, UK

Mary Lou Spitz, St Joseph Mercy Hospital, Pontiac, Michigan, USA

Hans Troidl, Universität zu Köln, Cologne, Germany

Joseph M Weerts, Clinique Saint Joseph, Liège, Belgium

Stephen White, Hospital Saint Roch, Nice, France

Foreword

The involvement of general surgeons in endoscopic techniques and now, exciting laparoscopic therapeutic manoeuvres, reflects a worldwide phenomenon that has not only brought surgeons closer together, but has also created an explosion which has manifested itself by the application of minimal access techniques to classic general surgical problems. All of this excitement and global interaction is manifested in this book, edited by David Rosin. The contents reflect a wide-ranging and diverse application of laparoscopy as presented by innovative and thoughtful surgeons who have now taken traditional 'open' surgical procedures and adapted them to safe and appropriate uses for the laparoscope.

This latest addition to Radcliffe Medical Press' series on minimal access medicine and surgery will set a standard for surgical description in the area of minimal access techniques. Although, from an historical perspective, minimal access surgery is in its infant stages, the technology and creative use of modern techniques have set a pattern of future discovery and enlightening evolution which will indeed be the standard for general surgery in the future. The wealth of information and foundation for future development encompassed in this book bodes well for all of us involved in the global excitement of endoscopic surgery.

Frederick L Greene
Professor of Surgery
University of South Carolina School of Medicine
January 1994

Preface

'*He who is prepared to ignore the past must be prepared to repeat it.*'
George Santayana

The excitement engendered by minimal access surgical techniques continues unabated, especially in the field of general surgery. Although general surgery remains the foundation on which other surgical specialties are based, it was one of the last to embrace minimal access techniques.

However, the speed at which general surgical operations have been performed by video-enhanced telescopic minimal access surgery has been phenomenal. This is recognized by the chapters included in this book which demonstrate the skill and ingenuity of the authors. They have all contributed to the development of minimal access surgery and their experience is even greater now than when they wrote their chapters. Their pioneering work has helped make these operations standard procedures.

Laparoscopic cholecystectomy exploded onto the general surgical scene like no other procedure before it. Embraced by the public and promoted by technological advances, it has rejuvenated general surgery. Although there were a few sceptics, the rush to learn minimal access surgical techniques was extraordinary and took surgical trainers by storm. Training is a very important topic and we must ensure standards are maintained.

Once again, I should like to thank Andrew Bax, Gillian Nineham, Kate Martin and all at Radcliffe Medical Press Ltd who have produced, with the help of the contributors to whom I shall always be indebted, a magnificent second volume in the series.

'*It is astonishing with how little reading a doctor can practise medicine, but it is astonishing how badly he can do it.*' William Osler.

R David Rosin
January 1994

History

DAVID ROSIN

Surgery is as old as mankind. Surgery is an art of working with the hands. Its name derives from the Latin word *chirurgia*, which in turn comes from the Greek *cheiros* ('hand') and *ergon* ('work'). In previous times, surgery in general and general surgery were synonymous. In the latter half of the twentieth century, general surgery has become more specialized, almost by default, as the surgical specialties have developed and broken away from it. These other specialties have evolved along anatomical divisions, eg urology, neurosurgery and orthopaedic surgery.

A definition of general surgery was given by the sixteenth-century French surgeon Ambroise Paré: *'The five duties in surgery: to remove what is superfluous, to restore what has been dislocated, to separate what has grown together, to reunite what has been divided and to redress the defects of nature.'* Nowadays this definition no longer holds, as general surgery really deals with gastrointestinal disorders and abdominal wall problems. In small communities and many general district hospitals, however, where specialization has not occurred to the same extent as in teaching hospitals, general surgery still includes vascular, endocrine and oncological surgery, as well as surgery of the gastrointestinal system and the abdominal wall.

The single most important factor limiting the work of early surgeons was their lack of anatomical knowledge. Today, anatomy is having to be relearned as a result of the different views of parts of the body obtained by video-enhanced telescopic surgery. Nowhere is this more true than in the surgery of inguinal hernia.

One of the best authorities on Greek medicine is a Roman encyclo-paedist of the early first century AD, Aulus Cornelius Celsus. In his *De Medicina*, he went into great detail regarding some surgical remedies. In the *Prooemium* of Book 7, he wrote: *'The third part of the art of medicine is that which cares by the hand . . . it does not omit medicaments and regulated diets (the other two parts of medicine), and does most by hand. The effects of this treatment are more obvious than any other kind.*

Inasmuch as in diseases, since luck helps much, and the same things are often salutory and often of no use at all, it may be doubted whether recovery has been due to medicine or a sound body or good luck ... But in that part of medicine which cures by hand, it is obvious that all improvement comes chiefly from this, even if it be assisted somewhat in other ways. This branch, although very ancient, was practised more by Hippocrates, the father of all medical art, than by his forerunners ....

'*Now a surgeon should be youthful, or at least nearer youth than age; have a strong and steady hand which never trembles; an ability to use the left hand as well as the right; with vision sharp and clear, and spirit undaunted; and be filled with pity, so that he wishes to cure his patient, yet is not moved by his cries, to go too fast, or cut less than is necessary. He does everything just as if the cries of pain cause him no emotion.*'

Again it is interesting that in Hippocrates' time, a two-handed surgical technique was regarded as important. This is now well recognized in minimal access surgery. Although useful in conventional open surgery, it is not as vital as in video-enhanced telescopic surgery.

The fact that surgery is based on anatomical knowledge was well founded and avidly pursued in the School of Alexandria in Hellenistic times. However, it was removed from the medical curriculum and only reinstated in the sixteenth century due to the interest in the human form shown by artists such as Leonardo, Raphael, Donatello and Michaelangelo. A further development which enhanced understanding and knowledge of anatomy was the invention of printing. At last illustrations, so necessary for anatomical study, could be accurately reproduced and distributed.

The history of surgery in the eighteenth century saw the development of modern pathology and experimental surgery, both associated with the name of John Hunter. The medical historian, Fielding H Garrison, gave Hunter a fitting epitaph: '*With the advent of John Hunter, surgery ceased to be regarded as a mere technical mode of treatment, and began to take its place as a branch of scientific medicine, firmly grounded in physiology and pathology.*' The influence of John Hunter continued in the first half of the nineteenth century. Hunter had made sure that all his students had a thorough grounding in anatomy, physiology and surgical pathology. Sir Astley Cooper, perhaps the most eminent London surgeon of the first part of the nineteenth century, was one of his pupils and a very fine operator. No doubt this was in part due to his devotion to anatomical study which he practised and taught in his private dissecting rooms.

However, despite Hunter, his students and their advances, there were numerous obstacles blocking the advance of surgery. Pain, infection, haemorrhage and shock were four of the most difficult to overcome. As each was dealt with, the boundaries of surgery expanded, and individual surgeons became more and more specialized. The discovery and use of anaesthesia made surgery painless and increased its scope. In 1842, a rural Georgian practitioner, Crawford W Long, used ether to remove small skin tumours, although he did not report this use until three years after William Morton had successfully anaesthetized a patient using ether at Massachusetts General Hospital on 16 October 1846. Chloroform was introduced the very next year by James Young Simpson of Edinburgh, and a new age in surgery was born.

Although anaesthesia found speedy acceptance, the same was not true for the attempts made at controlling infection. Pus in a wound was called 'laudable', in that once it had discharged, wounds healed, albeit slowly. Semmelweis and Oliver Wendell Holmes had shown in the 1840s that puerperal fever was carried to women in labour on the hands of their doctors. Simple washing in chlorinated lime solutions was extremely successful on Semmelweis' wards, but his Viennese colleagues paid little heed to his findings. It was left to Lister to convince the world that wound infection was evil, not laudable, and that it could be effectively prevented.

Despite anaesthesia, the development of many new techniques and the promise of antisepsis, John Eric Erichson (one of the most influential and perceptive surgeons of late nineteenth-century Britain) stated in 1873: *'There must be a final limit to development in surgery there can be no doubt . . . like every other art, be it manipulative, plastic or imitative, it can only be carried to a certain definite point of excellence. An art may be modified, it may be varied, but it cannot be perfected beyond a certain attainable limit. There cannot always be fresh fields for conquest by the knife; there must be portions of the human frame which will ever remain sacred from intrusion, at least from the surgeon's hands. That we have nearly, if not quite, reached these final limits there can be little question.'* However, the story of the past hundred years has proved Erichson to be a poor prophet.

Among the many difficult technical problems faced by nineteenth-century surgeons, was that of reconnecting the divided ends of hollow tubes, especially blood vessels and intestine. The basic principle of intestinal suture, that the serous coats should be brought into contact, was not discovered until the early nineteenth century and not put into use until some decades later. Furthermore, it was not until the German and German-trained surgeons began putting antiseptic and aseptic principles to work that the techniques of abdominal surgery found their way into common practice. While surgeons were learning to operate on tubular structures, so did the development of looking into these tubes develop.

The development of endoscopy

There were three phases in the development of endoscopy:

1   the rigid phase from 1805–1932
2   the semi-flexible phase from 1932–57
3   the fibre-endoscopy phase from 1957 to the present.

The oldest forerunner of the modern endoscope was devised by Phillipe Bozzini[1], an obstetrician who practised in Frankfurt am Main and who developed an instrument for seeing into the bladder and rectum with candlelight reflected by mirrors (Figure 1.1). It was demonstrated to the Alert Faculty in Vienna, who rejected it as a 'magic lantern', and it was apparently never put into practice. Antonin J Desormeaux[2] developed an alcohol lamp and lens system (Figures 1.2 and 1.3), but although the endoscope reached the stomach, the light source was insufficient. Instead it was used to view the urinary bladder, cervix and uterus.

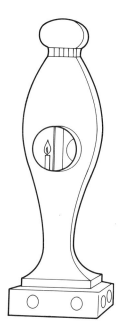

Figure 1.1: Bozzini's cystoscope consisting of a lamp, mirror, and candle. (Reprinted with permission of J.B. Lippincott & Co.)

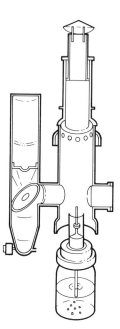

Figure 1.2: Desormeaux's endoscope incorporating kerosene lamp, mirror, and chimney vent. (Reprinted with permission of J.B. Lippincott & Co.)

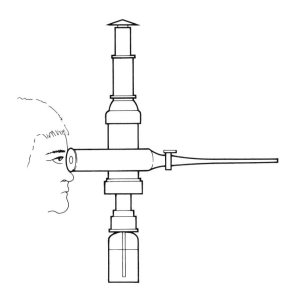

Figure 1.3: The Desormeaux endoscope used as a cystoscope in 1853. (Reprinted with permission of J.B. Lippincott & Co.)

The first internal light source was invented by Bruck, a dentist from Breslau, who, in 1867, examined the mouth of a patient using an electrically plated platinum wire as the light source. As there was a risk of burning the tissue, he later developed a water jacket for cooling the platinum wire. It was not until Edison invented the incandescent light bulb in 1880, and the Germans improved optical systems in the 1890s, that endoscopy became a practical procedure.

The first gastroscope was introduced by Adolf Kussmaul in 1868, apparently after watching a sword-swallowing exhibition.

In 1897, Max Nitze, a urologist from Berlin, produced the first usable cystoscope with lenses and electric lighting (Figure 1.4). He was helped by a German optician, Beneche, and a Viennese electro-optician, Joseph Leiter. A few years later, in 1901, Kelling reported using a cystoscope to inspect the peritoneal cavity of a dog after insufflation with air. He then coined the term 'celioscopy' to describe this technique. At this time, cystoscopy and other open-cavity endoscopic procedures (eg oesophagoscopy, proctoscopy and laryngoscopy) were well established[3].

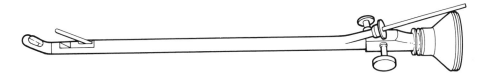

Figure 1.4: The Nitze cystoscope showing bulb illuminator and ureteral probe through probe channel. (Reprinted with permission of J.B. Lippincott & Co.)

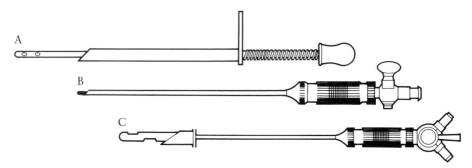

Figure 1.5: Insufflation needles. A: Goetze needle for induction of pneumoperitoneum. B: Verres needle to induce pneumothorax. C: Semm modification for monitoring of intra-abdominal gas pressure. (Reprinted with permission of Springer-Verlag.)

'Closed-cavity' procedures had not yet been tried, but the stage was set for the development of laparoscopy. In 1910, a Swedish surgeon, Jacobaeus, performed the first laparoscopy and thoracoscopy in a human[4]. He is credited with coining the terms 'laparoscopy' and 'thoracoscopy'. The importance of pneumoperitoneum was recognized a short time later, and prompted Goetze to introduce his insufflation needle in 1918. In 1938, Verres of Budapest wrote about his insufflation needle for producing a pneumothorax[5]. This needle is still used today (Figure 1.5). The first laparoscopic lysis of adhesions was performed by Fervers in 1933, and Boesch of Switzerland is credited with the first tubal sterilization in 1936[6,7].

The development of instruments

Meanwhile, in 1881, Johann Von Mickulicz-Reddecki developed an instrument which could be angled by 30° near its lower third. During the next 50 years, improvements in electric light sources, ocular systems and photographic methods resulted in the creation of more advanced instruments. In 1952, Rudolph Schindler introduced a new semi-flexible gastroscope based upon the optical principle proposed by Lang in 1917. He had discovered that clear images could be transmitted by a series of convex lenses around a gentle curve, provided that the curvature was not too great.

In 1930, Heinrich Lamm demonstrated that fine threads of glass fibre could be bundled together to act as a conduit for a light source, and that the bundle could be flexed or bent without losing its transmission capabilities. No-one knows why the idea languished for nearly 25 years, but it was in 1954 that the most significant advance was made by Harold H Hopkins and N S Kapany, who pointed out the potential application for endoscopy (Figure 1.6). Hirschowitz and his group created the prototype three years later, a genuine breakthrough in the examination of the oesophagus, stomach and duodenum.

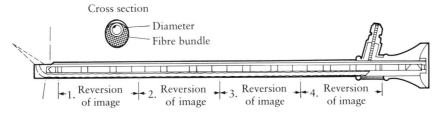

Figure 1.6: Cross section of laparoscope showing Hopkins' rod-lens system (and fibre-optic light illumination). (Reprinted with permission of J.B. Lippincott & Co.)

The first instruments provided a lateral view and used a distal electric bulb as their light source. Subsequent modifications have provided the practitioner with a straightforward (0°) view, while the lateral viewing device is now reserved for special examinations. Changes in light source from the distal electric bulb to the external light unit, and sophisticated light-conducting fibreglass bundles, eliminated excessive heat production and occasional burns caused by the distal light bulb in the stomach.

Prior to using insufflation, the introduction of an endoscope through the abdominal wall had been associated with many major and minor complications. There was a risk to the underlying bowel and vascular structures, which still exists despite insufflation. In 1946, Decker introduced an alternative method by inserting the laparoscope into the abdominal cavity through the cul-de-sac of the vagina, because of the dangers to underlying structures during laparoscopy, and named the procedure culdoscopy.

In 1944, Raoul Palmer in Paris stressed the importance of monitoring intra-abdominal pressure[8]. However, it was another 20 years before Kurt Semm in Kiel, Germany, developed an automatic insufflation device that monitored abdominal pressure and gas flow[9]. Previously air had been introduced into the peritoneal cavity by means of a syringe. With the development of safe insufflation needles, as well as instruments for controlling gas flow during pneumoperitoneum, complications were significantly reduced. However, because laparoscopy was considered a 'blind' procedure, with the risk of injury to intraperitoneal structures, acceptance was slow throughout the world.

Laparoscopy

Diagnostic laparoscopy was performed by many gynaecologists but only a few general surgeons. It was the gynaecologists and urologists who breached the frontiers of minimal access surgery during the second half of this century. Surgeons in both these specialties soon added operative skills to this minimal access approach for diagnosis. Semm must take much of the credit for the development of laparoscopic instruments such as needle holders, microscissors, clip applicators and atraumatic forceps.

Laparoscopic visualization of the peritoneal cavity was once restricted to the surgeon, and participation by other members of the team was limited. Therefore complicated operative procedures proved to be tedious because of the inability of assistants to interact with the surgeons. Articulated attachments containing a series of mirrors could split the image from the instrument, but these proved to be inefficient and cumbersome.

In 1986, this problem was solved with the development of the computer-chip TV camera which could be attached to instruments. Thus began the era of video-guided surgery. Elaborate developments in the area of video imaging resulted in high-resolution video monitors, affording greater clarity and definition as well as improved magnification of the operative field, and making fine dissection more simple.

General surgery

It is interesting to look back at the development of many operations in general surgery which have become so much simpler since the last century. The natural progression has been to inflict 'less and less damage' to our patients, and minimal access surgery is a further development along these lines. Taking a few examples, the operation for treatment of duodenal ulcer has changed dramatically: from partial gastrectomy introduced by Billroth in 1881, to antrectomy, then to total vagotomy and a drainage procedure, which in turn was modified to selective vagotomy with drainage, then to highly selective vagotomy or proximal gastric vagotomy. The development of these operations means that they have become more physiological and less invasive, but they have all needed a laparotomy to enable the surgeon to perform them. The healing of the patient, especially after operations such as highly selective vagotomy, was really only related to the laparotomy wound.

The advent of effective medical treatment made these operations less frequent, but now that they can be performed using video-enhanced telescopic surgery, through tiny incisions which do not take any time to heal and do not debilitate the patient, a review is needed to look at how duodenal ulcers should be treated. Many patients find it difficult to be compliant with medical treatment, and indeed the cost of a highly selective vagotomy via the minimal access route is probably very much lower than medical treatment which has to continue for more than a year.

Laparoscopic cholecystectomy totally transformed this operation. Cholecystectomy was first introduced by Langenbuch in Berlin in 1882, and proved to be an excellent operation, but again a large incision was necessary to ensure safe access. Patients were kept in hospital, merely because of the laparotomy wound and not because of the removal of their gallbladder.

The introduction of laparoscopic cholecystectomy, which was first performed in 1986 by the German surgeon Mühe and then recorded in 1987 by the French surgeon Philippe Mouret, has made this operation probably easier for the surgeon and certainly more friendly for the patient[10,11]. Since then it has become the established method of removing the gallbladder and has allowed the whole surgical team to see the operation rather than just the principal surgeon. It has opened the way to many other minimal access general surgical procedures and really put video-enhanced telescopic surgery on the map.

A faster recovery, less discomfort and earlier return to full activity has meant that video-enhanced telescopic surgery is now being used for virtually every intraperitoneal operation. It has proved useful in appendicectomy, where wound infection has been decreased and recovery has been faster, despite the fact that conventional appendicectomy is carried out via a very small incision. Laparoscopically-assisted operations such as in colonic surgery have greatly reduced the time spent in hospital, and ileus is less likely to occur due to the fact that the intestine is not handled.

One of the problems that still confronts surgeons performing minimal access surgery is the removal of bulky tumours. However, the fact that much mobilization can be performed without a large incision, using minimal access techniques, has shortened hospital time and made patients' recovery more rapid. There is no doubt that in reparative operations when no specimen is resected (eg in hiatus hernia repair, vagotomies and hernia repair) minimal access techniques have transformed surgery. Patients are much more willing to undertake these operations, knowing that they will be in hospital for shorter periods and will not experience the pain which results from a large incision.

Hernia repair

The history of hernia repair is fascinating, as the early part is really the history of the discipline of surgery. Many developments in the knowledge of hernia anatomy and treatment occurred during the eighteenth century. Sir Percival Pott refuted many of the old theories concerning the aetiology of hernia, and many of the methods of treatment based on these theories. He was probably the first surgeon to suggest the congenital origin of hernia. Once again, the treatment of hernias depended very much on knowledge of anatomy. Early in the nineteenth century, four men contributed significantly with descriptions of the inguinal anatomy: Camper, Cooper, Hesselbach and Scarpa all contributed to our knowledge.

The pure anatomist Sir Astley Cooper published his two-volume work *The anatomy and surgical treatment of abdominal hernia* in 1804 and 1807. First descriptions attributed to Cooper include transversalis fascia, internal ring, inguinal canal, correct formation of femoral sheath by the transversalis fascia and a complete description of Camper's fascia. He paid little attention to the 'ligament of the pubis', now called Cooper's ligament. He certainly had no idea of how important this structure would become in the modern treatment of hernia.

Edoardo Bassini devised a reconstruction technique of the inguinal floor with transposition of the cord. This operation included high ligation of the sac and reinforcement of the floor of the canal by suturing the conjoined tendon to the inguinal ligament beneath the cord, thus placing the cord under the external oblique aponeurosis. William Halsted in the United States developed an operation similar to that of Bassini almost simultaneously. The only difference was that in the Halsted operation the cord was transposed above the external oblique aponeurosis.

The importance of the posterior inguinal wall in the aetiology, as well as the repair of hernias, was recognized relatively late. Over the last 40 years a nylon darn at the shouldice repair have been recommended by a number of surgeons.

Much more recently, however, Lichtenstein showed that a tension-free repair using a mesh proved to have a very low recurrence rate[12]. This repair was not popular in Europe, where the introduction of foreign materials was not common in inguinal hernia repairs. However, it was soon realized that a tension-free repair was more physiological. The fact that the mesh could be placed into a preperitoneal pocket, using video-enhanced telescopic surgery with minimal access, made this type of repair even more attractive. The anatomy of the region had to be relearned, as its appearance from inside is very different from the anatomy encountered via the conventional approach. The diagnosis of indirect inguinal hernia is definite on laparoscopy, and the ability to treat bilateral hernias through tiny incisions is of great benefit. Thus minimal access surgery once again is the latest development in a long line of hernia repairs.

The future

Looking back on all that has happened in the history of surgery, it may seem impossible to predict what will happen next. Success will result from being able to balance available resources in terms of science, technology and personnel and solve problems as they change with time. We face a potential or certain increase in many such problems, and surgery will have to develop in order to catch up with them.

Sophisticated medical equipment is perhaps the first sign that surgery – which began as a manual of skill – has matured into an integral aspect of science and technology. The advent of virtual reality will make minimal access surgery seem antiquated in the not-too-distant future. For the moment, however, minimal access surgery is the greatest advance this century.

References

1   Bozzini P (1806) Lichtleiter, eine Erfindung Zur Anschung Innerer Theile und Krankheiten Nebst Abbildung. *J. Pract. Arzeyhunde.* 24:107.

2   Desormeaux AJ (1865) Transactions of the Société de Chirurgie, Paris. *Gazette des Hop.*

3   Kelling G (1901) Uber Oesophagoskopies, Gastroskopie und Colioskopie. *Munch. Med. Wochenschr.* 49:21–4.

4   Jacobaeus HC (1910) Uber die Moglichkeit, die Zystoskopie bei Unteruchung seroser Hohlungen anzuwenden. *Munch. Med. Wochenschr.* 57:2090–2.

5   Verres J (1938) Ein neue Instrument zur Ausfuhrung von Brust oder Bauchpunktionen und Pneumothoraxbehandlung. *Deutsche Med. Wochenschr.* 64:1480–1.

6   Fervers C (1933) Die Laparoscopie mit dem Cystoskope. Ein Beitrag zur Vereinfachung der Technik und zur Endoskopischen Strangdurchtrennung in der Bauchole. *Med. Klinik.* 29:1042–5.

7   Boesch PF (1936) Laparoskopie. *Schweiz A. Krankenhaus Anstaltsw.* 6:62.

8   Palmer R (1947) Instrumentation et technique de la colioscopie gynécologique. *Gynecol. Obstet.* 46:422.

9   Semm K (1989) History. In: Sanfilippo JS and Levine RL *et al.*, eds. *Operative gynecologic endoscopy.* Springer-Verlag, New York.

10   Mühe E (1986) Die erste cholecystektomie durch des laparoskop. *Lagenb. Arch. Chir.* 369:804.

11   Mouret G (1991) From the first cholecystectomy to the frontiers of laparoscopic surgery: the future perspectives. *Dig. Surg.* 8:124–5.

12   Lichtenstein IL, Shulman AG, Amid P and Montller MM (1989) The tension-free hernioplasty. *Am. J. Surg.* 157:188–93.

2

General Principles

CHRISTOPHER RUSSELL AND SARAH CHESLYN-CURTIS

Minimal access or minimally invasive therapy has changed surgical thinking in a manner which has surprised the cynic of just a few years ago. Minimal access surgery came about partly as a result of developments which took place in the late 1970s, when therapeutic endoscopy was beginning to change management. For example, the advocates of endoscopic sphincterotomy for stones in the common bile duct were discussing 'no-scar' surgery. Other teams were considering the use of endoluminal fibre-optic instruments to diagnose, biopsy and cauterize accessible tumours. Radiologists were beginning to assess intra-cavity pathology with the aid of improved imaging through the use of ultrasound and computed tomography (CT) scanning and to biopsy abnormal tissues and drain collections of fluid or pus.

In 1984 a percutaneous procedure study group was established at The Middlesex Hospital. By then, urologists had already started percutaneous nephrolithotomy[1], and extracorporeal shockwave lithotripsy was being evaluated for gallstone destruction[2]. The undoubted value of intra-abdominal abscess drainage by percutaneous techniques was leading to a re-evaluation of the management of traditional surgical areas, and the improved ability of conservative therapy to deal with conditions such as acute diverticular problems without open surgery was setting the scene for changing surgical attitudes.

The progress being made by our gynaecological colleagues, however, seemed to have little impact on general surgical thought, despite several studies confirming the advantage of diagnostic laparoscopy in the management of the acute abdomen. Even the clear description of laparoscopic appendicectomy by Semm in 1983 failed to stimulate the general surgeon.

The start of the minimally invasive therapy revolution for the general surgeon was undoubtedly the first cholecystectomy performed by Philippe Mouret in the Spring of 1987 in Lyon. When a nurse challenged Professor Dubois, saying that his mini-cholecystectomy incisions were too big, Dubois visited Mouret in Lyon; his subsequent work in the pig enabled him to undertake the first laparoscopic cholecystectomies during 1988.

Definition

Minimal access surgery is defined as the achievement of a therapeutic objective by the least physiologically disturbing stimulus so that the metabolic, cardiorespiratory and psychological effects are minimal. The therapist must weigh the risks of the minimally invasive technique against the benefit achieved by the lack of physiological disturbance. The removal of a stone from the common bile duct by dilatation of the sphincter of Oddi using an endoscopic approach, provides an excellent example of the advantages of minimally invasive surgery. The surprising feature of minimal access surgery is that it is the trauma of access, eg through the abdominal incision, which appears to excite the various physiological responses.

Irrespective of terminology, minimal access surgery is invariably performed from a distance with long, fine and specially designed instruments, which are introduced into the body either blindly into a pre-formed gas-containing cavity or under radiological control. The operation itself requires some kind of imaging – radiological, ultrasound guided, endoscopic or video – and the operator must not proceed after the initial puncture unless vision is clear enough for the instruments to be placed in the desired position. Mistakes in minimal access surgery often occur because the imaging is inadequate, which places much emphasis on the equipment available. In all forms of minimal access surgery the operator may not have full three-dimensional images and hand/eye co-ordination must be developed to a greater degree than would be necessary with traditional surgical techniques.

Minimal access surgery encompasses the various assisted operative procedures whereby, with imaging techniques or laparoscopy, a surgical component of the procedure can be much reduced in severity: in laparoscopy-assisted vaginal hysterectomy, for example. A surgeon can use imaging to locate a tumour (eg an adrenal tumour) accurately, and to approach it using specially designed retractors and instruments so that the lesion can be removed through a 3–4 cm incision. The definition of minimal access surgery may also include various oesophageal procedures which are undertaken either by endosurgical techniques or transthoracic coelioscopic surgery in conjunction with gastric mobilization and which can greatly reduce trauma.

The essence of minimal access surgery is to re-examine surgical techniques and to determine how procedures can be altered by use of modern equipment to reduce the physiological disturbance to the patient, and so enable the patient to recover more quickly.

Scope of surgery

As currently practised, minimal access surgery encompasses five approaches.

- Laparoscopic surgery includes cholecystectomy, vagotomy, repair of hiatus hernia, splenectomy, adrenalectomy, appendicectomy, hernia repair and resection of colon.

• Endoluminal surgery includes sphincterotomy, injection of ulcers and varices, excision of intestinal tumours, and laser dilatation of oesophageal cancer and rectal cancer.

• Perivisceral endoscopic surgery includes oesophagectomy and nephrectomy.

• Thoracoscopic surgery is now broadening its scope: cervical sympathectomy is the commonest procedure, followed by vagotomy, mobilization of the oesophagus, ligature of bullae and pleurodesis.

• Intra-articular surgery includes meniscectomy and removal of foreign bodies from joints.

In addition to these primary surgical approaches, there are the mixed radiological surgical procedures (such as percutaneous cholecystolithotomy) and the pure radiological procedures (such as the insertion of a drain into an abscess cavity).

Criteria for evaluation of minimal access surgery

With the increasing enthusiasm for minimal access surgery there is a danger that the achievement of a particular surgical procedure by a laparoscopic or alternative approach may gain such prestige that traditional surgical principles are laid aside. Minimal access surgery must always be balanced against the traditional procedure so that an evaluation can be made about the advantages and disadvantages. For instance, if the procedure is incomplete by minimal access surgery or breaks the basic surgical principles (such as in the Lichtenstein hernia repair) then it is obvious that the traditional approach is better. If the operation takes an excessively long time to perform, its cost-effectiveness must be called into question. Similarly, if there is no reduction in the hospital stay or in the length of time before full normal activities can be resumed, there may be little point in undertaking minimal access closed surgery. However, direct comparisons are hard to make. Minimal access surgery requires new skills that may be difficult for the older surgeon to learn. Furthermore, the number of operations that have to be performed before competence is attained appears to be greater with minimal access surgery than with traditional techniques; and many surgeons have found that they are still learning after 50 or 100 operations.

Many patients opt for the minimal access procedure as a result of the good publicity which it has received, and remain unaware of the disadvantages. This may lead to a poorer outcome unless the surgeon is vigilant. For instance, despite the trend towards undertaking colonic surgery laparoscopically, there is some doubt that it is effective against cancer in the long term.

The standard way of comparing old and new treatments is to undertake a controlled clinical trial. Unfortunately, ethical restraints and resistance by patients and surgeons have limited the investigator's ability to offer a random choice of operation to patients. With gallbladder surgery, for instance, few patients will accept randomization for laparoscopic or mini-cholecystectomy, so full comparison of these two therapies cannot be undertaken. A system of comprehensive surveillance seems to be the only realistic option at a time when laparoscopic procedures are spreading. This continued surveillance should be maintained at a level which will allow long-term evaluation of both the old and new procedures, and an extensive computer-based databank should be established. Any new procedure should be part of a continuing multi-institutional audit[3].

Thus any surgeon undertaking minimally invasive surgery must provide full and careful documentation of each procedure. His records should be good enough to allow comparison between the new procedure and the traditional technique. By comparing outcomes, complications and the lengths of time in hospital and before returning to work, it should be relatively easy to show that laparoscopy is preferable to traditional surgery. It is particularly important, when dealing with operations for cancer or those procedures with high recurrence (such as vagotomy or the surgical management of oesophagogastric reflux), that follow-up is maintained to assess the long-term effectiveness of the procedure. The danger is that the procedure may give such technical satisfaction that the surgeon loses awareness of the operation's objective, namely the long-term health of the patient.

Techniques in minimal access surgery

Minimal access surgery is a co-operative effort in which several teams of therapists may be involved in the management of a particular patient. Specialism will inevitably be marked and it is unwise to think that one person can be endoscopist, radiologist and surgeon.

Radiological approach

The radiologist offers two services in minimal access surgery. The first is to undertake a biopsy under radiological control, preferably using the Biopty gun. Such specimens can be large enough to provide tissue for proper histological techniques including immunohistocytochemistry. The second is to use guidewires, to dilate a tract so that a drain or an Amplatz sheath can be inserted. A tract can then be developed to allow the extraction of stones or debris and the drainage of an abscess or fluid collection. Abscess drainage is now a major part of the armamentarium of the radiologist and there is considerable evidence to show that abscess drainage by means of percutaneous technology is better than that provided by open operation[4]. This technique of percutaneous access and the establishment of a tract in conjunction with balloon dilatation can be used to dilate strictures.

The value of stone removal by percutaneous cholecystolithotomy remains to be fully evaluated, but in the approach to the intrahepatic biliary stone this technique probably surpasses all other methods[5]. In the occasional patient who has the misfortune to have a stone stuck in the intrahepatic biliary tree, often in its own pouch, access via the sphincter of Oddi is very difficult, even with a so-called 'baby scope'. Easier access can be achieved by passing a drain into the dilated intrahepatic duct and dilating the track so created to a size compatible with the passage of a 9 or 11 French flexible choledochoscope. Such an instrument will enable the endoscopist to see the stone, apply a lithotripsy stimulus such as electrohydraulic shock wave or a laser beam to disrupt the stone, and so enable the stone to be removed in fragments with flushing from above through a previously opened sphincter of Oddi.

Endoscopic approach

With the current enthusiasm for laparoscopic techniques, the role of the endoscopist in minimal access surgery has become underestimated. Nevertheless, endoscopists were the first to develop no-scar surgery. At present, endoscopy of the upper or lower intestinal tracts can remove polyps, biopsy ulcers or tumours, cauterize bleeding lesions, enable the injection of vessels and the division of sphincters, such as the sphincter of Oddi, to allow endoscopic removal of biliary stones.

Balloon dilatation under direct vision by means of an endoscope has yet to be fully evaluated; it has a role in the management of stenotic lesions, but its long-term effect is open to debate, particularly concerning strictures of the biliary tree. The use of the laser to remove large areas of tumour can provide most satisfying palliation for those dying as a direct result of their tumour.

The endoscopist is now entering a further surgical field with the development of techniques for the passage of tubes into the intestine or stomach to create a jejunal or gastrojejunal feeding access. Similarly, lesions adjacent to the intestinal tract can now be approached safely through the wall of the intestinal tract; such examples are the draining of a pseudocyst through the wall of the stomach or the duodenum.

The role of endoanal surgery has yet to be evaluated but it does seem that this technique is of value in the excision of a tumour of the rectum and that adequate clearance of a submucosal lesion in the elderly patient can be achieved by this form of surgery.

Laparoscopic approach

Many optimists and advocates of the laparoscopic technique consider that laparoscopic surgery (or preferably coelioscopic surgery) has few bounds. Nevertheless, the procedures at present in general use appear to be those most likely to stand the test of time. Laparoscopic appendicectomy is reasonably straightforward and allows a speedy recovery and early return to activity. Laparoscopic cholecystectomy has similar advantages and is undoubtedly the procedure that is most logically performed laparoscopically.

The reason for these two operations being ideal for the laparoscopic

approach is that they are excisional procedures and there is minimal reconstruction required. Within the abdomen or any other abdominal cavity it
appears that it will be easy to excise lesions but always difficult to reconstruct.
Suturing will remain tedious and time-consuming, lacking the accuracy that is
so necessary for complex anastomoses, unless some form of stapling device to
create a join or anastomosis or repair of structures can be developed, which is
simple enough to be handled down a laparoscope.

With patience, more extensive intra-abdominal procedures can be undertaken, such as vagotomy, removal of liver cysts and the common gynaecological procedures. The removal of larger organs such as the spleen or colon
presents problems to the laparoscopist because of the sheer physical size of
these organs and the difficulty of removing them from the abdominal cavity.
However, the advent of an impermeable bag and morcellator may well
overcome this problem and lead to the ability to remove an intra-abdominal
structure completely without leakage of cells into the abdominal cavity which
is always a problem with cancer surgery.

Colonic surgery will undoubtedly come to be a major component of
laparoscopic techniques. Various ways of dealing with the colon, either
through small incisions or delivery through the rectum, are currently being
evaluated. Similarly, anastomotic techniques either inside or outside the
abdomen have been developed to introduce the topic of laparoscopically
assisted procedures. Perhaps vaginal hysterectomy aided by the laparoscope
is the most logical area for such a procedure. The abdominal operator must
ensure that the major parts of the operation, during which structures such
as the ureter can be damaged, are dealt with under direct vision rather than
blindly as with the perineal approach. If the best way to ensure minimal access
to the patient is to combine an open and closed technique, then that is entirely
acceptable.

Surgical approaches

It is frequently forgotten that the concept of minimal access surgery can apply
to the open operation. The tradition of making large incisions came about as a
result of inadequate surgical instrumentation and anatomical knowledge: the
surgeon and assistant had to be able to get their hands into the wound in order
to perform surgery.

Techniques now enable the whole operation to be done at a distance using
long instruments, and the dissection to be done with instruments like the hook
diathermy which are accurate and do not obscure the view of the surgeon. The
hook diathermy also enables a bloodless field to be maintained. For instance,
a splenectomy can be performed through a small wound provided that the
splenic artery is tied well before the splenic vein to allow the blood from the
spleen to suffuse out through the draining splenic veins, so decreasing the size
of even a large spleen. By using muscle stretching techniques, for instance with
the gridiron incision in appendicectomy, destruction of muscle fibres can be
reduced so that the pain of the incision is minimal and metabolic disturbance
is subsequently reduced.

The performance of a procedure should not be compromised by a small approach because minimal access surgery depends upon using good retraction, good lighting and a good technique to provide ideal vision and thereby to perform a procedure that is undoubtedly safer than traditional surgical techniques.

Most of this book relates to laparoscopic techniques and therefore subsequent technical discussions will be confined to the laparoscopic approach.

General principles of laparoscopy

Preoperative preparation

All patients should be fully informed that a laparoscopic operation still constitutes a surgical procedure. The patient should also be warned that there are potential complications such as significant haemorrhage, bowel perforation or other visceral injury. In case of such an emergency, permission for a laparotomy should be specifically given in order to control complications and facilitate a difficult procedure so that the operation becomes a laparoscopic assisted intervention.

For most operations, it is reasonable to give a single dose of antibiotic prophylaxis. If the gastrointestinal tract is in any way compromised during the procedure, however, or if during a cholecystectomy or appendicectomy the organ is opened or pus is released, then a wide-spectrum antibiotic should be given for a further two or three doses according to severity of contamination.

Prior to the operation, patients should be screened for blood antibodies and the blood group should be determined. The general fitness of the patient requires careful assessment and no operation should be undertaken unless both the surgeon and the anaesthetist consider that the patient is fit for it. Most laparoscopic procedures are more comfortably performed under a general anaesthetic, although heavy sedation can be used for certain pelvic procedures such as sterilization or simple diagnostic laparoscopy.

Creation of a pneumoperitoneum

The Verres needle has been used in laparoscopy since 1938. It consists of a hollow blunt obturator inside a sharp trocar which allows safe introduction into the peritoneal cavity. The surgeon should check that the instrument is correctly assembled and flushed to ascertain patency. The site of election for introduction will be determined by previous surgery, but it is most frequently below the umbilicus – since this is the thinnest part of the abdominal wall – or at either iliac fossa lateral to the lateral edges of the rectus abdominus muscle. It is important to hold up the abdominal wall when introducing the needle to allow the abdominal contents to fall away.

This procedure can be performed by placing a Kocher forceps on either side of the skin incision near the umbilicus. After the needle is introduced, opening the tap and holding up the abdominal wall will produce a hiss which confirms the position of the needle in the peritoneal cavity. Other tests are to aspirate and inject saline to ensure that the needle is not in a blood vessel and to use the 'hanging drop' technique. None of these tests is 100% accurate but when combined they do help to reassure the operator that the needle is correctly placed. If blood is aspirated the needle must of course be withdrawn and reinserted. If bowel injury occurs, the injury should be assessed. The injury may be repaired under laparoscopic control, if the operator is proficient, or dealt with by open surgery. A minor visceral injury may be treated conservatively[6].

A number of gases have been used to create the pneumoperitoneum, but carbon dioxide is the most frequent choice. Certain problems are associated with this gas, such as depression of pH and elevation of carbon dioxide tension, vascular collapse and intense vasodilatation giving the appearance of peritonitis. Some operators maintain that nitrous oxide is less painful, but the length of laparoscopy and the abdominal pressure maintained are more likely to blame for the right shoulder-tip pain which results from diaphragmatic stretching and phrenic nerve stimulation.

Insufflation should initially commence at no greater than 1.5 l/min since it has been demonstrated in the dog that this is the maximum amount that can be tolerated if the vena cava is inadvertently punctured. In addition, with careful monitoring of the patient, it is easier to spot cardiac dysrrhythmia or hypo- or hypertension so that there is ample warning of problems and insufflation can be ceased.

Before starting a laparoscopic procedure, it is essential that the surgeon is familiar with the laparoscopic insufflator to ensure that correct pressures are used. After creation of the pneumoperitoneum it is important to determine which trocar should be inserted. It is easier to insert 5 mm trocars but the telescope accommodated through the small trocar sheaths does not transmit enough light and the image is not bright or magnified enough for detailed surgical procedures. When inserting the trocar it is important to use the left hand as a break to prevent sudden deep penetration which would inadvertently injure intraperitoneal or retroperitoneal structures. Furthermore, the trocar should be aimed away from the aorta.

If the patient has had previous surgery, it may be difficult to create a pneumoperitoneum. It is safer to make a slightly larger periumbilical incision and make an incision in the linea alba under direct vision, incise the peritoneum and insert the trocar under direct vision. The insufflation can then proceed and the pneumoperitoneum be created with perfect safety[7].

Throughout these manoeuvres it is ideal to keep the intraperitoneal pressure at no more than 15 mmHg, although pressures up to 25 mmHg can be tolerated for short periods. Close co-operation with the anaesthetist to ensure adequate ventilation is important with the higher pressures.

Insertion of telescope and working ports

The 0° or 30° 10 mm laparoscope is inserted through the trocar sheath and the peritoneal cavity inspected. Correct placement of the laparoscope is the first objective and therefore the surrounding bowel and tissue are inspected to ensure that no damage has occurred as a result of the insertion of the first trocar. The remaining abdominal viscera should be visualized systematically. Much of this initial inspection should be performed with the video monitor. As the peritoneal cavity is inspected it is important to determine the best places for the other ports, which should be inserted under direct vision to limit the possibility of damaging other organs[8].

The siting of the ports depends upon the operative procedure to be performed. It is essential that the working ports provide an adequate angle between the operating instrument and the holding instruments so that traction can be exerted in the appropriate directions in order to facilitate easy dissection. Additionally, it is important when placing the ports to avoid the epigastric vessels; these can be transilluminated and avoided.

Laparoscopic instrumentation

A wide variety of instruments is available, but usually the fewer the instruments involved the better[9]. Perhaps the most important instruments are those used for holding the organ such as the gallbladder. Such instruments should have teeth which grasp but do not penetrate and therefore do not slip and tear during the traction.

Throughout the procedure it is important to be gentle and to avoid excessive pressures. Blunt dissection should be avoided as this tends to tear vessels and create bleeding. Careful scissor dissection or hook diathermy should be used at all times so that a dry field is maintained as far as possible. This is aided by an irrigation suction device which should enable high volumes of fluid to be inserted and sucked out. To prevent clotting of the fluid within the tube, a heparinized saline irrigating solution (7500 units/l) is helpful. When vigorous suction is being used it is easy to lose the pneumoperitoneum; this is prevented by short bursts of suction and as far as possible sucking beneath the fluid level. High-volume insufflators are essential for most dissection and these should be set to the automatic high-flow position to maintain an adequate pneumoperitoneum.

Electrosurgical principles

Diathermy is crucial in laparoscopic dissection to maintain a field free from blood[10]. This has led to a re-examination of diathermy and an awareness of the different characteristics of monopolar and bipolar instruments and high frequency versus electrocoagulation for dissection. High-frequency monopolar cutting diathermy is dependent on the production of electric arcs concentrating the entire continuous unmodulated current onto a single point where the tissue is immediately vaporized. The operating peak voltage to produce this effect is in the range of 200–500 V. Tissue cutting is not achieved if the voltage drops below 200 V. Above 500 V the electric arcs produced are of such intensity that the tissue is carbonized and the electrode is damaged.

Within the safe operating range, the depth of the coagulation of the cut edges increases with increasing voltage and intensity of the electric arcs. It is also influenced by the thickness of the cutting electrode and the rate and depth of the movement by the operator. With an impedance of 250 Ω, fluctuations in the current on the output voltage and intensity of the electric arc are produced by variations in the depth and rate of cutting. This disadvantage can be overcome by automatic control circuits with sensor electronics. This ensures that the intensity of the electrics is kept constant irrespective of the speed and depth of the cut. For the operator it is important that the voltage is reduced to the minimum in order to avoid cutting beyond the area coagulated so that bleeding is not increased by the technique. The setting on the machine must be adjusted to limit injury to the surrounding tissues.

Electrocoagulation is produced by a modulated current; when applied, the temperature in the tissue rises in proportion to the resistance of the tissue, the duration of current flow and the square of the root mean square of the electric current density. Because of different tissue characteristics the temperature rises at different rates and subsequent charring can make division of the tissue difficult, necessitating cutting as opposed to further coagulation. It cannot be overemphasized that the particular characteristics of the diathermy machine must be understood so that the current is controlled throughout.

Some of the problems associated with monopolar diathermy can be overcome with bipolar electrocautery, in which the heating of the tissue is confined to the area between the two ends of the probe and the current does not flow through the patient. Only minimum power is necessary and safety is thus ensured. Bipolar hooks, loops and forceps are now available but they require frequent cleaning because of the coagulum which forms on the surface.

Laser coagulation

There has been considerable debate and controversy regarding the relative benefits of laser versus electrocoagulation in laparoscopic surgery[11]. Although the matter has not been entirely resolved, most now favour electrosurgery. The four lasers commonly used in laparoscopic surgery are argon, Nd:YAG, KTP and Ho:YAG. KTP deploys a crystal of potassium titanyl phosphate to frequency double a beam of Nd:YAG to green light. Most laparoscopic laser dissections are carried out using the contact mode rather than the free beam mode because of the enhanced safety and the tactile feedback.

A specific major disadvantage of lasers during laparoscopic dissection is the risk of inadvertent damage from the overshoot phenomenon whereby the laser energy penetrates through the intended target and damages deeper structures. Unintentional damage may also be inflicted by perfect beam columnation and shake in the non-contact mode. Claims that less smoke is generated by laser than by electrocautery are largely unsubstantiated[12].

Ligation of structures

A perceived difficulty in laparoscopic surgery has been the inability to control bleeding and close open structures without the use of suturing[13]. These problems have been largely overcome by the use of metal clips to secure the cystic duct, for instance, or the appendix stump and arteries. Unfortunately, the metal which is left behind can interfere with subsequent imaging procedures, and there is also a possibility that the clip will not completely occlude the vessel, giving rise to leakage from the cystic duct stump. Often the instruments for applying the clips are clumsy and difficult to position accurately. However, new instruments have a better facility for rotating the clip applier once in the sheath, and absorbable clips of polydioxone (PDS) are now available so that there is no foreign body left behind after the procedure.

Despite the use of convenient clips it is appropriate for the would-be laparoscopist to learn knots which can be applied within the abdomen. The preferred technique is the slip knot, first described by Roeder for use during tonsillectomy and adapted for use in pelvic laparoscopic surgery by Semm. This knot can be tied outside the abdomen and then slipped by a push rod to lock firmly in place around the stump of the appendix, cystic duct or vessel. Special catgut has proved to be the only appropriate material and now specially prepared pre-knotted sutures are commercially available.

If the use of the Roeder loop and knot makes the pedicle too wide for easy tying, then the commercially available stapling machines are extremely useful: they can place three layers of staples and divide between the layers if appropriate. This will undoubtedly extend the range of laparoscopic colonic surgery as well as facilitating other procedures. Finally, the laparoscopist must be practised in the art of intra-abdominal suture. This requires patience and care and an understanding of the limitations of a two-dimensional image in a three-dimensional cavity.

Complications

In a large series of gynaecological laparoscopic operations the mortality rate was reported as 0.03%. Other studies suggest that the mortality approached zero with minor and major complication rates of 4% and 0.6% respectively[14]. Absolute contraindications to laparoscopic surgery are intestinal obstruction, generalized peritonitis, abdominal wall infection and coagulopathy which cannot be controlled by blood products. Relative contraindications include obesity, ascites, a large umbilical hernia and a previous abdominal operation that would create significant adhesions preventing the formation of an adequate pneumoperitoneum.

Properitoneal or omental emphysema is the most significant problem that may arise during Verres needle insertion and insufflation of carbon dioxide. If properitoneal insufflation is not recognized early the peritoneal membrane will be markedly distorted, resulting in poor identification of normal anatomical landmarks. Similarly, insufflation of carbon dioxide into the greater omental apron may cause this structure to bloom and prevent location of other peritoneal structures. Nevertheless, with patience these collections rapidly absorb. The Verres needle is small and therefore puncture of the intestine or a vascular structure will cause only minimal injury and should not cause problems provided that it is recognized.

Tension pneumoperitoneum will result if the carbon dioxide insufflation pressure is greater than 30 mmHG. Resulting respiratory or circulatory difficulties will be observed by the anaesthetist. This complication can be found most commonly in obese patients in whom the weight of the abdominal wall is such that a good pneumoperitoneum cannot be created without higher pressures. It is important that a good insufflation machine be used with a safety setting preventing continued insufflation when the pressures rise to higher levels.

Complications at the time of trocar and sheath insertion are usually a result of technical error or anatomical abnormalities. The most dreaded injury is puncture of the abdominal aorta or other related arterial or venous structure. The injury may become rapidly evident on insertion of the laparoscope. Initial management would be to leave the laparoscopic sheath in position and then proceed to an emergency laparotomy. The trocar sheath unit is not removed until the vessel is fully exposed and controlled, because the trocar acts to tamponade the bleeding.

Injury to the deep epigastric vessels is recognized early in the procedure due to constant dripping of blood into the abdomen along the sleeve. In many cases, this can be managed by coagulating the parietal peritoneum around the trocar. Failing this manoeuvre, the abdominal wall should be incised medial and lateral to the sheath down to the peritoneal membrane. Suture ligatures are then placed on either side of the blood vessel.

Injury to the bowel by the trocar and sheath should be evaluated by open exploration. However, if the surgeon is particularly skilled and the damage is minimal, appropriate suturing can prevent contamination. Careful postoperative observation is indicated in such circumstances and a laparotomy should be performed if there is evidence of continued peritoneal contamination.

Injury to the bladder can be managed by a Foley catheter.

Problems which arise during the laparoscopic procedure itself are most usually related to haemorrhage. Prevention of haemorrhage is the prime principle of laparoscopic surgery. When haemorrhage occurs, pressure is the appropriate management. If the vessel is occluded by pressure for several minutes it will usually stop bleeding for long enough to allow the clip to be placed accurately. Blind application of the clips, particularly around the porta hepatis, is known to give rise to injury of vital structures such as the common bile duct. It is preferable to open the patient rather than to persist with multiple clip application.

Postoperative management

Following a laparoscopic procedure, the patient should wake up promptly with minimum discomfort and pain. If a nasogastric tube has been inserted during the operation to remove excess intraluminal gas then this should be removed prior to waking. Postoperative discomfort can be prevented by the insertion of a diclofenac suppository and injecting bupivacaine (Marcain) around the laparoscopic puncture wounds, particularly the umbilical incision.

The patient is encouraged to mobilize early and fluids can be given within two or three hours of the operation. At this stage, the abdomen is most difficult to assess as it tends to be distended and tender. Nevertheless, if the patient's condition is not satisfactory, vigilance is required to ensure that there is no intra-abdominal bleeding or leakage of gastrointestinal contents. Repeated clinical examination is the appropriate management technique. Ultrasound is invariably misleading as the gas prevents good visualization. Occasionally CT scanning may be necessary if there is a real dilemma. Provided that the field is dry at the end of the procedure, haemorrhage is unlikely; if it does occur the usual parameters of pulse, blood pressure and lowered venous pressure are good guides. Operative intervention is appropriate if there is real doubt.

A common postoperative effect is shoulder-tip pain. It is still difficult to determine the origin of this pain but it is said to be related to stretching or irritation of the diaphragm by fluid collecting around the liver. Some have tried to prevent the pain by aspirating all the gas at the end of the operation or injecting a local anaesthetic into the peritoneal cavity. No specific manoeuvre can be guaranteed to relieve the discomfort, which the patient can usually accept once the condition has been explained to them. Most patients will be able to leave hospital within a few days of laparoscopy.

Long-term complications are few and these are related to wound problems. Wound infections should be uncommon. Unfortunately if they do occur, particularly in the umbilicus, they can lead to local sepsis and early development of an incisional hernia. By careful attention to wound infection and to closing the linea alba (which is apt to split), these complications can be avoided.

Laparoscopic surgery provides significant advantages over open procedures, but safety remains paramount and any unnecessary risk jeopardizes the good reputation of this surgery. A careful audit of complications is essential to ensure that the morbidity and mortality of laparoscopic procedures remain well below the rates for open operations. The key to safety is adequate training[15] and a proper understanding of the apparatus and the technique.

References

1   Amplatz K and Lang PH (1986) *Atlas of endourology.* Year Book Medical Publishers, Chicago.

2   Sauerbruch T, Delius M, Paumgartner G *et al.* (1986) Fragmentation of gallstones by extracorporeal shock waves. *N. Engl. J. Med.* **314**:818–22.

3   Neugebauer E, Troidl H, Spangenberger W *et al.* (1991) Conventional versus laparoscopic cholecystectomy and the randomized controlled trial. *Br. J. Surg.* **78**:150–4.

4   Hemming A, Davis NL and Robins E (1991) Surgical versus percutaneous drainage of intra-abdominal abscesses. *Am. J. Surg.* **161**:593–5.

5   Koo Han J, Choi BI, Park JH and Han HC (1992) Percutaneous removal of retained intrahepatic stones with a pre-shaped angulated catheter: review of 96 patients. *Br. J. Radiol.* **65**:9–13.

6   Yuzpe AA (1990) Pneumoperitoneum needle and trocar injuries in laparoscopy. *J. Reprod. Med.* **35**:485–90.

7   Jarrett JC (1990) Laparoscopy: direct trocar insertion without pneumoperitoneum. *Obstet. Gynecol.* **75**:725–7.

8   Winfield HN, Donovan JF, See WA *et al.* (1991) Urological laparoscopic surgery. *J. Urol.* **146**:947–8.

9   Cuschieri A (1991) Minimal access surgery and the future of interventional laparoscopy. *Am. J. Surg.* **161**:404–7.

10   Hunter JG (1991) Laser or electrocautery for laparoscopic cholecystectomy. *Am. J. Surg.* **161**:345–9.

11   Watson G (1992) What can lasers really do? *Min. Inv. Ther.* **1**:173–8.

12   Cuschieri A (1992) Laparoscopic treatment of gallbladder disease. *Min. Inv. Ther.* **1**:115–23.

13   Nathanson LK, Easter DW and Cuschieri A (1991) Ligation of the structures of the cystic pedicle during laparoscopic cholecystectomy. *Am. J. Surg.* **161**:350–60.

14   Ponsky JL (1991) Complications of laparoscopic cholecystectomy. *Am. J. Surg.* **161**:393–5.

15   Bailey RW, Imbembo AL and Zucker KA (1991) Establishment of a laparoscopic cholecystectomy training program. *Amer. Surg.* **57**:231–6.

3

Laparoscopic Cholecystectomy

J. PERISSAT, D. COLLET, M. EDYE, R. BELLIARD, J. DESPLANTEZ AND E. MAGNE

Born in secret in 1987, and developed in an atmosphere of scepticism and hostility throughout 1988, laparoscopic cholecystectomy (LC) triumphed in 1989 and 1990 and caused a veritable revolution in the world of general surgery. The 777 consecutive cases that we report reflect the spirit of these various periods. From being conservatively restrictive, our indications widened to include 90% of gallstone cases. For us, the sclero-atrophic gallbladder still constitutes the greatest endoscopic challenge, and should be reserved for the most experienced operators. The figures for mortality (0.13%) and complications (3.3%), which include three common duct injuries (0.4%), are comparable to, if not better than, those for traditional cholecystectomy. The quality of recovery is markedly better: virtual absence of pain, short hospitalization, return to normal physical activity within ten days, rapid return to work and preservation of the abdominal musculature in those who play sports. These advantages are unavailable to the 5.5% of patients for whom an intraoperative conversion to an open procedure is necessary. Their recovery is that of traditional cholecystectomy, which itself is far from being poor. The large multicentre studies such as those carried out in France and Belgium recently, reporting 3708 cases, have arrived at identical conclusions. LC is set to become the gold standard for treatment of gallstones and is the first step towards surgical techniques of the twenty-first century which will be performed inside the musculocutaneous envelope of the unopened human body.

We started our laparoscopic approach to gallstones in November 1988, and had performed our first 100 cholecystectomies by December 1989[1]. Since then, new instruments have become available, new results have been published and numerous teams have started working in the field. By September 1991, we had carried out 777 consecutive laparoscopic cholecystectomies. The aim of this chapter is to report the results of these procedures and describe the evolution of our indications and operative technique.

The patients

From November 1988 to September 1991 we offered LC to 777 patients (*see* Table 3.1). These patients are a mixed group, spread out over a period of time, during which our selection criteria and operating techniques evolved. The patients can be divided into three groups.

Group I was made up of our first 104 patients. Since we were in practically unknown territory, we deliberately selected patients suffering from uncomplicated biliary colic for this new procedure, to the exclusion of those with acute cholecystitis or a history of numerous previous inflammatory attacks. We also excluded pregnant women and patients with common bile duct (CBD) stones and cardiorespiratory risk factors, however small. We did not eliminate obese patients. Figure 3.1 summarizes our selection criteria.

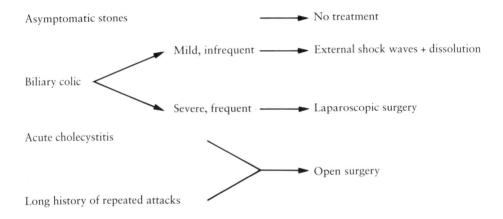

Figure 3.1

	N	%
Age: 13 to 83 years		
Sex: 582 females, 195 males		
Mortality	1	0.1
Laparotomy conversion	43	5.5
Complications	26	3.3
CBD injury	3	0.4

Table 3.1: 777 patients operated on with laparoscopic cholecystectomy between November 1988 and September 1991.

The preoperative investigation included a cardiorespiratory assessment, a hepatic assessment with hepatic function tests based on cholestasis (bilirubin, transaminases, alkaline phosphatase, gamma-GT), ultrasonography of the liver and biliary tract and intravenous cholangiography (IVC) with tomography. If duct visualization was poor (with obese patients in particular), endoscopic retrograde cholangiopancreatography (ERCP) was performed. This group of patients covered our activity from November 1988 to December 1989.

Group II was made up of 617 patients. The only absolute contraindications were the existence of an unstable cardiac state or previous upper abdominal surgery affecting the stomach, liver or pancreas.

In this group, 161 patients were operated on semi-urgently for acute cholecystitis; 63 of them had a long history of bouts of acute cholecystitis treated medically. None of these patients presented with symptoms, either in the past or more recently, that might have suggested the presence of CBD stones although we looked routinely for the presence of asymptomatic stones.

Preoperative workup was the same as for group I except that cholangiography was performed only in specific circumstances. If ultrasound showed a CBD calibre of 8 mm or more, ERCP was performed. If ultrasonography was normal but the hepatic function tests showed abnormalities (elevated alkaline phosphatase or gamma-GT), IVC with tomography was performed, except in the case of an overweight patient in whom it could have been misleading, and on whom we performed an ERCP.

Group III was made up of 56 patients who were referred for treatment of gallstones and whose principal symptoms were the presence of CBD stones. All patients had stones in the gallbladder.

These patients had the same cardiorespiratory and hepatobiliary function assessments as the preceding group I and II patients and, in addition, all underwent ERCP.

Evolution of operative technique

Instrumentation

This has varied somewhat from our first publication, because of the arrival of a number of new instruments[1]. We now prefer to use an axial vision laparoscope, either at 0° or 30° for the laparoscopy.

For dissection, haemostasis and control of the cystic duct, we continue to use an electrocoagulation hook which uses monopolar current with variable intensity, mixing cutting and coagulating current. We also use bipolar diathermy.

We tend to use scissors increasingly for dissection. We no longer use Filchee clips, preferring the use of titanium clips. The automatically rechargeable clip-applicators mean a considerable gain in time and operating comfort.

When the gallbladder contains stones larger than 10 mm, intracorporeal lithotripsy is usually required, the gallbladder either being left in place or detached from its bed and partially withdrawn through the umbilicus. So as to avoid the loss of small particles of calculi into the peritoneal cavity during these manoeuvres, we sometimes use what we call the 'bag extraction' technique, with a sterile, resilient plastic bag which is rolled up and inserted through a 10 mm cannula. The bag is unfolded inside the abdomen and the stone-containing gallbladder is placed in it. The bag should be strong enough to remain intact when firmly grasped and pulled through the abdominal wall. If extraction is not possible, an ultrasonic lithotriptor or stout forceps is inserted into the bag to break up the calculi and evacuate them separately, thus reducing the size of the bag so that it can be easily removed.

The instrument tray should include a catheter directing forceps to help cannulate and secure the cystic duct for operative cholangiography. One or more endoligatures should also be available for closure of the cystic duct stump if it is friable due to inflammation and clips are likely to cut through.

The operation

The surgeon stands between the supine patient's outstretched legs. The layout of equipment and positioning of operating staff remains identical to previous descriptions[2] when we performed intracorporeal lithotripsy with the aid of two assistants (*see* Figure 3.2). With a small team (a single assistant), the TV screen is placed to the right of the patient, the assistant to the patient's left and the scrub nurse to the patient's right. An articulated bracket holding the laparoscope and camera can be used instead of a second assistant.

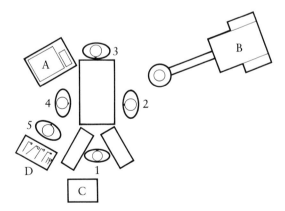

Figure 3.2: 1: Operating surgeon 2: First assistant 3: Anaesthesiologist 4: Second assistant 5: Scrub nurse
A: TV screen, insufflator and light source B: X-ray machine C: TV screen for X-ray D: Instrument table

Insufflation of the peritoneal cavity and insertion of instruments

Insufflation is commenced by puncture of the peritoneal cavity with a Verres needle in the left hypochondrium about 3–4 cm from the costal margin in the mid-clavicular line where adhesions are seldom found. Once the peritoneal cavity has been filled with carbon dioxide to a pressure of 8–12 mmHg, the needle is swept in an arc under the abdominal wall to check that the umbilical region is free. If so, the laparoscope is introduced through the umbilicus by means of a cannula 10 mm in diameter. If not, another insertion point through a clear zone higher up in the midline must be found.

The various instruments for grasping, irrigation, suction and dissection are then introduced (*see* Figure 3.3). We prefer this placement because it permits us to work with the penetration axis of the instruments at a right-angle to the visual axis. Moreover, inserting the dissecting instrument through the left hypochondrium enables elevation or depression of a large left liver lobe.

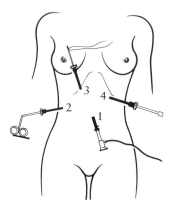

Figure 3.3: 1: Laparoscope 2: Grasping forceps 3: Irrigation cannula 4: Hook dissector, scissors and clip applier

The elevation of the inferior surface of the liver by the irrigation-aspiration device and the upward and outward pull of the claw forceps inserted through the right hypochondrium enable better demonstration of the components of the triangle of Calot. This avoids pulling the cystic and common ducts in the same direction such as in a long cystic duct descending behind the common hepatic duct. If the cystic duct is short this prevents tenting of the CBD by excessive traction and inadvertent dissection or clamping of the cystic–common duct junction.

Dissection and control of the cystic artery and duct

Due to the way the instruments are arranged, as shown above, the right-hand forceps grasps the gallbladder fundus and pulls it upward and to the right, away from the duodenum and the CBD. An instrument inserted from the left (eg scissors, dissecting hook or grasping forceps) allows the connective tissues between the body of the gallbladder, the hepatic flexure and the duodenum to be divided and the cystic duct to be reached. Sometimes the cystic artery is reached first, especially when it is short, which prevents proper exposure of the triangle of Calot. Dissection here should be carried out with the scissors or the electrocoagulating hook without coagulation. Diathermy should be used sparingly close to the CBD due to the risk of aberrant conduction causing a full thickness burn to the duct wall which may present as a bile leak some days later. Control of the cystic artery or its branches should always be carried out close to the neck of the gallbladder and as far as possible from the CBD. Cannulation of the cystic duct for operative cholangiography should be performed after dissection, clipping and division of the cystic artery or its branches, the most perilous time for the CBD.

'Thou shalt not place any clamp nor divide any cylindrical structure without first being certain of its identity.' This golden rule of surgery in general applies equally to coelioscopic surgery. An intraoperative X-ray may be of help. If in doubt, the abdomen should be opened and the operation converted to traditional surgery.

Separation of the gallbladder from its hepatic bed is performed with the electrocoagulating hook or scissors. If the gallbladder is very distended, so that grasping it with forceps is hazardous or impractical, it should be punctured and aspirated, a bile specimen should be sent for culture and the gallbladder irrigated until clear. Thus, if the wall is breached during dissection, the risk of a later intraperitoneal sepsis is reduced. However, the puncture weakens the wall of the gallbladder and when the time comes for removal, it will tear or leak at the puncture point, showering stones into the peritoneal cavity.

Operative cholangiography

This is performed when preoperative imaging of the CBD is not possible or if the cystic duct appears to be larger than 2 mm at laparoscopy. At this diameter, stones may have migrated into the CBD and the catheter can usually be inserted more easily. If insertion into the cystic duct remains impossible after trying to dilate it with a balloon catheter, there is no point in persevering; we prefer to ligate the duct in a healthy area and not risk a split which could extend to the cystic–common duct junction and on into the CBD.

An X-ray can be used to detect a biliary leak at the point of dissection of the cystic artery or branches. This is one of the major arguments of those in favour of routine operative cholangiography.

We believe that this argument is questionable: either the CBD has been opened by mistake and it is unnecessary to wait for an X-ray to confirm it, or there has been a diathermy burn which is not visible on an operative cholangiogram. On the other hand, an intraoperative X-ray should be taken when recognition of the structures around the gallbladder neck is difficult. It is dangerous to attempt cannulation of a duct downstream from a clip without being sure that it really is the cystic duct. In this case it is better to perform a cholangiogram either by direct puncture of the gallbladder to determine the length and direction of the cystic duct or by fine needle injection of the CBD if the gallbladder outlet is occluded. The various well known anatomic anomalies of the biliary tract, always a pitfall for the surgeon, can thus be detected. In exceptional circumstances, if safe identification of the anatomy is impossible, the risk of damage to the CBD is such that we think it is wiser to perform a laparotomy.

Extraction of the gallbladder

There are three options, depending upon the circumstances.

- The gallbladder has solid walls and contains only a few very small stones. It is freed from its bed and extracted through the cannula in the left hypochondrium, the manoeuvre being viewed through the laparoscope inserted in the umbilical cannula.

- The gallbladder has very fragile walls due to inflammation or dissection. It contains large stones and will be difficult to extract. In this case we resort to the 'extraction bag' technique, as mentioned earlier. A large gallbladder containing very large stones can be opened inside the bag, the stones fragmented and the whole contents extracted.

- The gallbladder has resilient walls free of inflammation and contains large floating stones. Internal lithotripsy is performed with the gallbladder in place[3]. When the gallbladder is emptied of its calculous contents it is reduced to a small pouch which can be easily extracted through the sleeve of the cholecystoscope in the right hypochondrium.

Irrigation and drainage of the abdominal cavity

After extraction of the gallbladder, the position of clips on the cystic artery and duct is checked. Intensive irrigation is performed with isotonic saline solution at 37°C until the liquid is clear. With our first 100 patients we drained almost routinely with a sub-hepatic suction drain. At present we are much more selective and drain only in cases of gangrenous cholecystitis where the cystic duct is fragile or large and inflamed, and has been ligated as clips would not be reliable. After checking each puncture site for haemostasis, it is important to evacuate the pneumoperitoneum fully by depressing the valves of the cannulae, which are then removed. To minimize scarring, the 10 mm incisions are closed with a sub-cuticular stitch and all wound edges are neatly approximated with sterile adhesive strips.

Postoperative management

The operation is performed under general anaesthesia. All our patients remain in hospital at least overnight. The following day they can eat and walk normally. They are allowed to leave hospital at their own request and when we know that their family doctor will give them good medical follow-up at home. Many patients prefer to spend an extra night in hospital and return home on the second postoperative day. We advise a convalescent period of one week before resuming normal physical activity, and an additional week before returning to work. Some of the more active and highly motivated patients have returned to work a week after their operation.

Results

Table 3.2 summarizes the complications for groups I to III.

	Mortality	Conversion	Complication	CBD Injury
Group I (N = 104)	0	3	3	0
Group II (N = 617)	1	36	23	3
Group III (N = 56)	0	4	0	0
	1 (0.13%)	43 (5.5%)	26 (3.3%)	3 (0.39%)

Table 3.2: 777 patients operated on with laparoscopic cholecystectomy between November 1988 and September 1991.

Group I

In group I, mortality was nil[1]. We had to convert the laparoscopy into a laparotomy in three cases and there were three postoperative complications, none of which required open surgery.

In this highly selected group of patients, where the only symptom was biliary colic with no inflammatory features, either recently or in the patient's past history, the preoperative assessment detected asymptomatic calculi in the CBD in three cases. These were treated by endoscopic sphincterotomy prior to LC. The majority of patients had a sub-hepatic drain for 24 hours.

These excellent results, combined with the fact that we had gained in operating experience and that instruments more specific to coelioscopic biliary surgery had become available, enabled us to widen our indications (see Figure 3.4).

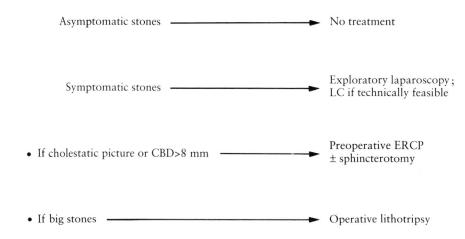

Figure 3.4

Group II

In group II there was one death, an 82-year-old woman operated on semi-urgently for acute cholecystitis who died without warning 48 hours after the operation while sitting in her chair. No autopsy was carried out and the cause of this sudden death remains unknown.

Conversion to open operation

We had to convert the laparoscopic procedure to an open operation in 36 patients (*see* Table 3.3.).

	Acute cholecystitis (N = 161)	Inflamed gallbladder (N = 63)	Non-infected gallbladder (N = 393)
Bleeding	3	3	3
Adhesions	4	10	1
CBD injury	1	1	0
CBD stones	3	0	1
Gallbladder perforation	1	0	0
Confusing anatomy	0	0	1
Equipment failure	1	0	3
	13 (8.1%)	14 (22.2%)	9 (2.3%)

Table 3.3: Reasons for conversion to laparotomy in 36 out of 617 group II patients.

It should be noted that 27 of these conversions took place in the group which presented with either acute cholecystitis or a gallbladder profoundly altered by previous bouts of inflammation (sclero-atrophic). The most frequent reasons for conversion were uncontrolled bleeding and dense adhesions around the gallbladder. There were four cases of bleeding of the cystic artery or branches, three cases of bleeding in the gallbladder bed and two cases where conversion was required due to the existence of portal hypertension secondary to cirrhosis undetected during the preoperative assessment.

The gallbladder can be buried under dense adhesions made up of the greater omentum, the hepatic flexure of the colon and the duodenum. As there is a significant risk of damaging the colon and/or the duodenum, dissection by electrocoagulation should be kept to a minimum and bipolar diathermy used if available. In 11 cases we abandoned the laparoscopic procedure because of the density of these adhesions. In four cases the dense hepatic attachments of an intrahepatic sclero-atrophic gallbladder caused us to beat a retreat.

Two injuries to the CBD occurred and were detected intraoperatively; one was lateral and there was one complete division where the CBD was mistaken for the cystic duct. A conversion to laparotomy enabled the first patient to be treated by insertion of a T-tube and the second by end-to-end repair.

In one case, an attempted lithotripsy with the gallbladder in place in a patient with gangrenous cholecystitis ended with multiple perforations of the gallbladder wall from the grasping forceps, from which stones escaped into the peritoneum. Laparotomy was necessary to terminate the cholecystectomy and completely lavage the peritoneal cavity. The postoperative course was uncomplicated.

Four cases of asymptomatic CBD stones led us to convert to laparotomy: on three occasions in an emergency procedure for acute cholecystitis where a thorough preoperative assessment had not been possible, and in one case where a stone suspected prior to surgery was confirmed by operative cholangiography. In none of these cases was it possible to remove the stone by transcystic laparoscopic techniques.

Complications

We had 25 postoperative complications in this group. Three required a second open surgical procedure. In one case a partial stenosis of the CBD was revealed due to a haemostatic clip on the cystic artery pinching and partially occluding the common hepatic duct. Because of the development of jaundice by the fifth postoperative day, the patient underwent reoperation to remove the clip. Although the compressed region showed a loss of wall thickness, there was no defect of the mucosa and we elected to insert a small T-tube. The postoperative course was uncomplicated. The second case was one of shock due to substantial bleeding two hours after LC in a patient with cirrhosis. Laparotomy and packing of the gallbladder bed was necessary to achieve haemostasis. The postoperative course was uneventful. The third patient developed an abscess in the pouch of Douglas necessitating a laparoscopy on the ninth postoperative day. The remaining complications are summarized in Table 3.4

	Acute cholecystitis (N = 161)	Inflamed gallbladder (N = 63)	Non-infected gallbladder (N = 393)
Bleeding	1	2	1
Bile leak	2	3	1
CBD stenosis	0	0	1
Intra-abdominal abscess	3	3	1
Acute pancreatitis	0	0	1
Acute ascites	1	0	0
Pyrexia of unknown origin	0	1	1
Other	1	2	1
	8 (5.0%)	11 (17.4%)	7 (1.5%)

Table 3.4: Postoperative complications in group II patients (26 complications in 617 patients = 3.7%).

We sorted the complications according to when they appeared after the operation, as shown in Table 3.5: early (within 48 hours), intermediate (from day two to day 20) and late (after day 20).

	Early	Intermediate	Late
Bleeding	1	3	0
Bile leak	2	3	0
CBD stenosis	0	1	0
Intra-abdominal abscess	0	5	2
Other 8	2	6	0
	5	18	2

Table 3.5: Appearance of postoperative complications in group II patients.

The early complications included major bleeding, mentioned above, and two biliary leaks adequately dealt with by the sub-hepatic drain placed at operation for acute cholecystitis. The spontaneous cessation of bile drainage after five to seven days following an initial flow of 400 ml per day prompted us to not pursue the origin of the leak which would have entailed an ERCP, itself not without risk.

A case of acute pancreatitis also occurred within 48 hours in a patient with microlithiasis of the gallbladder and a very narrow CBD with no stones evident on the operative cholangiogram. We are not certain for the reason for this episode, which settled on medical treatment.

The intermediate complications were bleeding, biliary effusions and intra-abdominal sepsis. Secondary haemorrhage was suspected when pain occurred about the fifth postoperative day after the patients had returned home. A significant anaemia and a sub-hepatic collection which showed on ultrasonography supported this hypothesis. We did not undertake treatment and the symptoms resolved spontaneously. Follow-up sonograms showed a small resolving sub-hepatic collection.

Three biliary effusions occurred as intermediate symptoms manifested by pain in the right hypochondrium and a fever between 37.5° and 38° C which appeared after a week without symptoms and after discharge from hospital. The effusion was diagnosed in all three cases by ultrasonography. In one, an ERCP showed a leak from the cystic duct stump where the clip was not tight enough. The CBD was dilated but showed no signs of calculi nor stenosis of the sphincter of Oddi, and the effusion was evacuated by means of an echo-guided puncture and positioning of a drain. There was no further biliary discharge and the drain was removed after 24 hours. In the second case, a further laparoscopy showed a sub-hepatic biliary effusion of which we were unable to find the origin and which resolved within a week with simple drainage. In the last case, a leak from the cystic duct resolved within a week by combining laparoscopically placed drainage and endoscopic sphincterotomy.

Five cases of intra-abdominal abscess in the sub-hepatic region appeared within ten days of the operation and after the patients had been at home for at least a week. The clinical picture was consistent: throbbing pain in the right hypochondrium accompanied by fever. The diagnosis was confirmed by ultrasonography and a leukocytosis. Treatment consisted of a second laparoscopy followed by the evacuation of the collected fluid, irrigation and insertion of a suction drain. Resolution occurred in 48 hours. All the patients had a straightforward recovery. Of these, four abscesses occurred after difficult cholecystectomy, one in a patient with acute cholecystitis and in three others after LC for a very inflamed sclero-atrophic gallbladder. In none of these cases had a drain been inserted during the operation.

The remainder of the intermediate complications in group II were more diverse: one bout of acute ascites in a cirrhotic patient two weeks after the cholecystectomy, and three general medical complications (heart failure, pulmonary infection and a fever which lasted ten days and then disappeared as suddenly as it had started).

Two patients developed an abscess in the pouch of Douglas which appeared on day 20 in one and day 24 in the other. The clinical picture was typical with pelvic pain and fever. The diagnosis was confirmed by ultrasonography. Both patients were treated by a second laparoscopy which enabled irrigation and drainage of the purulent fluid. Each abscess contained calculous debris which had escaped from the gallbladder at the time of its extraction. Such debris may not be as innocuous as some would suggest, but recovery was straightforward.

We should underline the fact that of the 26 complications in 617 patients treated, 19 appeared in the group of 224 patients operated for inflammation or acute cholecystitis.

Thirty-five clinically asymptomatic stones of the CBD were discovered in group II patients (*see* Table 3.6). In 28 cases they were discovered in the preoperative assessment. They were all treated by endoscopic sphincterotomy, generally prior to LC. In three cases the duct was cleared by endoscopic sphincterotomy during LC. Since the patients are supine, however, it is difficult to gain access to the papilla by duodenoscopy, so we shelved the idea of combining the two techniques.

In six cases we decided to do the LC first. A drain was secured in the cystic duct and endoscopic sphincterotomy was carried out two days after the LC. In seven cases the stone was found during the LC by operative cholangiography. In six of these cases the patients had undergone an emergency operation for acute cholecystitis and had not had a preoperative assessment. In the remaining case, the patient had undergone an elective procedure with no symptoms of cholestasis, and ultrasonography of the CBD was normal. Since the size of the cystic duct was more than 2 mm, intraoperative cholangiography was carried out which showed the stone.

In three cases we elected to leave the stone in place, to be extracted 48 hours later by endoscopic sphincterotomy. In the four other cases, using the same sequence of operation, we decided to convert the laparoscopy into a laparotomy in order to be able to treat a stone in the CBD by choledochotomy followed by a temporary transcystic drain.

Detected prior to LC	
Treated by ERCP + sphincterotomy	
Prior to LC	19
During LC	3
After LC	6
	28
Detected During LC	
ERCP + sphincterotomy	3
Conversion to laparotomy	4
	7

Table 3.6: Asymptomatic CBD stones in group II patients (35/617 patients = 5.6%).

A sub-hepatic drain was placed for 106 patients. In three cases a biliary effusion was transformed into a fistula and biliary peritonitis was thus avoided. Massive bleeding was detected rapidly in one case, leading to laparotomy. The six cases of intermediate or late intra-abdominal sepsis appeared in patients without a drain.

The patients with no complications or conversions to laparotomy had a recovery period free from pain and were able to resume normal physical activity less than a week after the operation. The average postoperative stay in hospital was 2.8 days (range 1–7 days). All the patients operated were reviewed four weeks after the LC, for those with no complications, and four weeks after the last procedure in cases with a complication requiring surgical or endoscopic treatment.

There was no evidence of medium-term complications. In this series, 132 patients were reviewed one year after the operation during a visit which included ultrasonography and the liver function tests mentioned earlier. No complications came to light, either locally (at the point of insertion of the cannulae) or at the biliary level (no residual CBD stones).

Group III

Group III was made up of 56 patients who all had clinical symptoms suggesting the presence of a stone in the CBD (*see* Table 3.7), either at the time of admission or shortly before (one to two weeks previously). Four presented with severe cholangitis without kidney failure and negative blood cultures. Of these, two had hyperamylasaemia, compatible with acute pancreatitis. All 56 patients underwent ERCP.

Abnormal liver function tests	55	
CBD dilatation or sonogram	48	
ERCP		56
CBD stones	43	
CBD clear	13	

Table 3.7: Clinical features of CBD stones in group III patients (N = 56).

In 43 cases we found a stone in the CBD associated with a dilated biliary tract and features of cholestasis. In one case the stone was situated in an undilated biliary tract with no signs of cholestasis. In seven cases with biochemical cholestasis, the CBD was dilated but free of stones. In six with biochemical cholestasis, the CBD was of normal calibre and free of stones.

We carried out 49 endoscopic sphincterotomies: in 43 patients in order to clear the CBD, and in six patients in order to open a papilla which was thought to be stenosed because of biliary tract dilatation in the absence of identifiable stones.

These 56 patients were to have an LC immediately after clearance of the duct. LC was performed in 32 cases the day after the endoscopic sphincterotomy, in nine cases on day two and in eight cases between days three and eight. For the remaining seven, sphincterotomy was performed for severe cholangitis and LC was deferred.

In four cases we elected to perform traditional cholecystectomy. In two cases the patients presented with hyperamylasaemia suggestive of acute pancreatitis at the time of onset of cholangitis. In one case there was a residual stone after the endoscopic sphincterotomy and we elected to remove it by choledochotomy during traditional cholecystectomy. In one case, since the ultrasonogram showed an empyema, we preferred to perform a traditional operation.

It should be stressed here that in none of the groups was a complication due to the pneumoperitoneum. Some authors report complications of 0.19% and greater.

Comments

By June 1991, our team had 32 months of practical experience of LC under its belt. Having originally gone into previously unexplored territory we were extremely careful about the selection of our first patients and carried out LCs only in the simplest of cases. Once we had reached our 100th patient, we expanded our indications so that the 40% of initial referrals considered contraindicated dropped to 18%. The results obtained in the first 104 cases were far better than those obtained by traditional cholecystectomy, but an assessment of our overall results shows that the figures and percentages of mortality and morbidity (*see* Tables 3.1 and 3.8) are almost identical to those obtained by traditional procedures (*see* Table 3.9).

The expansion of our indications meant that our rate of conversion to laparotomy increased from 3% to 5.5%. Postoperative complications remain stable (3% to 3.7%) but there were three lesions of the CBD and one death.

These results must be analysed in relation to the pathological state of the gallbladders removed and the level of our expertise at the time of LC.

		%
Mortality		0.13
Conversion		7.0
Morbidity		3.5
	Linked to conversion	0
	Linked to CBD	0.18
	Reoperation	1.2

Table 3.8: Mortality and morbidity in cholecystectomy by laparoscopic surgery in the Franco-Belgian series of 3708 cases (according to Testas *et al.*[7]).

		%
Mortality		0.5
Morbidity		4.2
	Linked to laparotomy	0.4
	Linked to CBD	0.1
	Reoperation	0.7

Table 3.9: Mortality and morbidity in cholecystectomy by open surgery (according to McSwain *et al.*[4]).

As for non-inflamed gallbladders (all of group I and the greater part of group II – see Table 3.2), the conversion rate remains essentially unchanged (3%, 2.3%). The rate of postoperative complications decreased by half (3% to 1.4%). This decrease is balanced by a higher figure for complications which appear when there is acute or chronic inflammation (such as sclero-atrophic gallbladder). It is in this last sub-group of patients that the highest percentage of complications occurred (11 out of 63 cases – 17.4%) and the conversion rate reached 22%. Do these results cast doubt on the advisability of LC in such patients? It is perhaps useful at this point to recall their clinical profiles: they have a long history of bouts of acute cholecystitis, with the gallbladder wall more than 4 mm thick, as shown by ultrasonography, and very little fluid around the stones. The best indicator remains the laparoscopic appearance showing dense adhesions around a very small gallbladder buried deep in the hepatic parenchyma.

In these circumstances, it is very difficult to define the triangle of Calot clearly and then to find a plane of dissection between the hepatic parenchyma and the gallbladder. In such cases, one should terminate the dissection of the cystic pedicle and revert to open surgery without a sense of failure. It is relatively easy to foresee these difficulties prior to the operation from the history and the sonogram. Patients should therefore be told that the likelihood of completing the procedure laparoscopically is 60–70%.

In the near future, we should see the rate of postoperative complications falling for this group of patients, at the price of an increase in the percentage of conversions which in turn will decrease as the experience of laparoscopic teams increases. We believe the cholecystectomy should at least begin with the exploratory laparoscopy, as two-thirds of such patients will benefit.

Indeed, it is the speed and comfort of the postoperative recovery that makes LC a major step forward. Usually there is no pain, the abdominal wall remains soft, digestive function returns quickly and normal physical activity can be resumed almost immediately. The disadvantages are more often than not associated with anaesthesia, causing nausea and sleepiness for a number of hours. Progress is needed in the choice of anaesthetic or in the avoidance of general anaesthesia altogether.

If rapid recovery after LC does not occur, complications should be suspected. These usually occur immediately or early in the postoperative period. Pain, tenderness of the abdominal wall, temperature and slight jaundice are all signs that should prompt immediate investigation either to prevent the complication or to treat it as rapidly as possible. The main examination techniques available are ultrasonography, CT scan, ERCP, white cell count and tests for cholestasis and cytolysis. Bleeding and biliary leaks can thus be detected.

One does not necessarily need to resort to open surgery to resolve these problems. Medication or a second laparoscopy is often sufficient. Even if postoperative recovery is a little prolonged, the patient has not lost the benefit of avoiding a large abdominal wound.

The excellent recovery from LC should also be available to patients with calculi in the CBD associated with gallbladder stones. If the stone in the CBD is clinically symptomatic, this should be treated first. Currently, endoscopic sphincterotomy after ERCP gives excellent results. Once the CBD is clear, an

LC is performed the following day or a few days later. Thus comprehensive treatment is available for gallstones, wherever they are located, by endoscopic means combining endoluminal endoscopy and laparoscopy.

Asymptomatic CBD stones should also be sought routinely. Progress in preoperative investigations is such that few stones are missed. Once the stone has been discovered, it must be removed by endoscopic sphincterotomy and the LC deferred a day or so. Our continued pursuit of asymptomatic CBD stones prior to LC is justified by the fact that it is not possible at present routinely to clear the CBD using laparoscopic techniques. In addition, in 5–10% of cases (depending on the operator's experience) it is technically impossible to carry out an endoscopic sphincterotomy. It would be detrimental to take the patient down the following path: laparoscopic cholecystectomy→discovery of an asymptomatic stone in the CBD that cannot be removed→failure of the subsequent endoscopic sphincterotomy→laparotomy, choledocotomy and removal of the CBD stone.

In this field, techniques are evolving rapidly and a standardized approach to CBD during laparoscopy will evolve in the near future. The advantages and disadvantages of this new technique must be evaluated and compared with those of endoscopic sphincterotomy which until now has given the best results.

New techniques which gain a place as rapidly in the therapeutic armamentarium as LC has done are few and far between. Following the initial reports of LC[5,6], over the past two years 3708 cases have been gathered in the surgical community in France and Belgium[7], as shown in Table 3.9. The results are very similar to ours (see Table 3.1). Similar tests are reported from other European countries[8,9], the USA[10–13] and Australia[14]. This is rightly called a revolution, for even if it is only a part of the trend toward less invasive surgery, it has tremendously accelerated change in the attitude of general surgeons to endoscopic techniques. We must lead this revolution which is essentially free of a negative side: by not resurrecting poor operations in traditional surgery simply because they can be performed laparoscopically[15]; by avoiding precipitous use of laparoscopic techniques without suitable training; and by appropriate analysis of the indications for their use. The group of patients with sclero-atrophic gallbladders, profoundly altered by previous bouts of inflammation, should remain in the hands of the best trained teams.

In the near future we shall see a profusion of publications reporting complications of LC and allowance must be made for a phase of technical maturation of the operators. The stakes are high, for the results of traditional cholecystectomy are already excellent. Each new operator should be determined to do at least as well as with traditional surgery from the outset by careful patient selection. Two to four years hence the average results will stabilize at the level of those already obtained by the pioneering teams.

Apart from educating surgeons in these techniques, there remains the problem of disseminating information to general practitioners and referring doctors. The length of the hospital stay for LC is short but complications can occur soon after discharge. Bleeding or major biliary leaks require a rapid and precise response and justify keeping the patient in or near the endoscopic surgery centre for at least 24 hours. Intermediate and late complications occur after a period free from symptoms and usually do not require urgent treatment. The role of the general practitioner or family doctor is vital so that complications can be detected and treated without delay. Some, such as biliary effusions, can hide behind insidious masks.

Other less invasive techniques for treating gallstones may be developed in the near future and we will then be able to fix precise limits to the indications for LC[16]. Currently, however, LC is becoming the standard treatment for gallstones in more and more institutions.

References

1   Perissat J, Collet D, Belliard R, Dost C and Bikandou G (1990) Cholécystectomie par laparoscopie. La technique opératoire. Les résultats des 100 premières observations. *J. Chir.* (Paris). **127**:347–55.

2   Perissat J, Collet D and Belliard R (1990) Gallstones: laparoscopic treatment – cholecystectomy, cholecystostomy and lithotripsy. Our own technique. *Surg. Endosc.* **3**:131–3.

3   Perissat J (1991) Gallstones: laparoscopic treatment – cholecystostomy, cholecystectomy and lithotripsy. *Dig. Surg.* Vol.8, No. 2:86–91.

4   McSwain GR, Prillaman PE, Johnson PA and Ganey JB (1986) Cholecystectomy: clinical experience with a large series: 1037 cases. *Am. J. Surg.* **151**:352–7.

5   Dubois F, Icard P and Berthelot G *et al.* (1990) Coelioscopic cholecystectomy: preliminary report of 36 cases. *Ann. Surg.* **191**:271–5.

6   Reddick FJ and Olsen DO (1989) Laparoscopic cholecystectomy. A comparison with mini-lap cholecystectomy. *Surg. Endosc.* **3**:131–3.

7   Testas P and Delaître B (1991) *Chirurgie digestive par voie coelioscopique.* Edition Maloine, Paris.

8   Cuschieri A, Dubois F, Mouiël J, Mouret P, Becker H, Buess G, Trede M and Troidl H (1991) The European experience with laparoscopic cholecystectomy. *Am. J. Surg.* **161**(3):385–7.

9   Troidl H, Eyrpasch E, Al-Jazini A, Spanberger W and Diehich A (1991) Laparoscopic cholecystectomy in view of medical technology assessment. *Dig. Surg.* **8**:108–13.

10 Berci G (1990) Coelioscopic cholecystectomy. *Ann. Surg.* **212**:649–50.

11 Reddick FJ and Olsen DO (1990) Outpatient laparoscopic laser cholecystectomy. *Am. J. Surg.* **160**:485–9.

12 Reddick FJ, Olsen DO, Spaw A, Baird D, Asbun H, O'Reilly M, Fisher K and Saye W (1991) Safe performance of difficult laparoscopic cholecystectomies. *Am. J. Surg.* **161**:377–81.

13 Zucker KA, Bailey RW, Gadacz TR and Imbembo AL (1991) Laparoscopic guided cholecystectomy. *Am. J. Surg.* **161**:36–42; discussion: 42–4.

14 Hardy K (1991) Percutaneous cholecystectomy. *Aust. NZ. J. Surg.* **61**:5–6.

15 Mouret G (1991) From the first laparoscopic cholecystectomy to the frontiers of laparoscopic surgery. The future perspectives. *Dig. Surg.* 8:124–5.

16 Cuschieri A (1991) Minimal access surgery and the future of interventional laparoscopy. *Am. J. Surg.* **161**(3):404–7.

4

Laparoscopic Laser Cholecystectomy

JOSEPH B. PETELIN

Removal of the gallbladder has remained the standard definitive treatment for symptomatic gallbladder disease for over 100 years. The procedure was first introduced in 1882 by Langenbuch, and although some modifications of the technique have occurred, the general conduct of the operation has been relatively unchanged. It has been routine to gain access to the gallbladder through the peritoneal cavity via an upper midline incision, a right subcostal incision, or a transverse upper abdominal incision.

In 1987, however, a new and revolutionary approach to gallbladder removal made surgical history, when Mouret and colleagues performed in that year, the first laparoscopic cholecystectomy in Lyon, France[1]. Rapid development of equipment and refinements of technique have characterized the short history of this new procedure. Whether performed with mechanical instruments such as scissors, with electrical instruments such as diathermy, or with more sophisticated tools such as lasers, the operation has been shown to be at least as effective as the standard open cholecystectomy, and much more beneficial to patients in terms of reduced pain, shortened hospital stay, and more rapid return to normal preoperative lifestyle[2-5].

This chapter explores this new operation with emphasis on the use of the laser as an energy source. It should be noted, however, that a number of energy sources may be used to complete the procedure; the laser itself is not the essence of the procedure. Rather, the essential features of the operation include

- the access route(s) to the operative site
- video enhancement of a telescopic image
- the use of a two-dimensional monitor to *guide* movements in a three-dimensional world
- the actual movements themselves, ie the technique.

Special emphasis will be given to performance of the operation using a single-surgeon two-hand technique.

Preoperative evaluation and patient selection

The clinical diagnosis of symptomatic gallbladder disease is usually based on historical findings of right upper-quadrant or epigastric abdominal pain which occasionally radiates to the interscapular region. Laboratory and radiographic investigations may include a variety of tests to evaluate liver function, gallbladder function (or dysfunction), and the presence or absence of gallstones or other pathology possibly related to the symptom complex[6]. It is not the purpose of this section to discuss the details of these preoperative tests. Suffice it to say that a standard battery of tests should be undertaken to document the diseased state of the gallbladder prior to consideration of its removal. In addition to these studies, suitability for general anaesthesia and possible laparotomy (in the event of conversion from the laparoscopic approach to the open method) should be determined by conventional means.

Patient selection is the next task for the general surgeon. The surgeon with little experience of laparoscopic cholecystectomy will have to apply more stringent criteria for selection of appropriate candidates than will be necessary after considerable experience has been gained.

Patients who have had previous abdominal surgery, and those who are severely ill, may not be the best candidates for the procedure unless the surgeon has well-developed laparoscopic skills[7-9]. Similarly, patients with known or suspected common duct stones will deserve special attention prior to laparoscopic cholecystectomy. In some cases, these patients may undergo endoscopic retrograde cannulation and sphincterotomy to clear common duct stones before laparoscopic cholecystectomy[10-14]. In other cases, and after significant experience has been gained, patients in this category may undergo laparoscopic cholecystectomy with laparoscopic common duct exploration[15-29].

The size of a patient's gallstone(s) does not really influence candidacy for laparoscopic cholecystectomy at any time, since stones as large as 7 cm have been successfully removed even by novice laparoscopic biliary tract surgeons. In fact, patients with large stones and relatively few stones are actually better surgical candidates for the less experienced surgeon, since these patients are less likely to have common duct stones, and if the gallbladder is accidentally perforated during dissection, it is easier to retrieve 'escaped' stones. Laparoscopic cholecystectomy during pregnancy remains controversial[30,31].

Finally, it is important to educate the patient properly about the procedure. Many patients have begun to think that laparoscopic cholecystectomy is 'minor' surgery since only small incisions are visible on the surface. They must understand that a general anaesthetic will probably be necessary and that there are very real operative risks similar to the open procedure, but that in most cases, there will be less pain, and they will be able to walk and be discharged from the hospital sooner than after open cholecystectomy. It is often important to educate the patient's family, and the nurses providing postoperative care, that it really is acceptable for the patient to feel good. Early in my experience, it was necessary to restrain nurses from administering narcotic analgesics as in the open procedure; in most cases only one or two doses of such medication are requested by the patient – quite different from the requirements of those undergoing open surgery.

Although it may still be controversial in some circles, it has been my practice to use some form of deep vein thrombosis (DVT) prophylaxis in all patients. Pulsatile anti-embolism stockings are used routinely. Subcutaneous heparin is used in high risk patients or those who have had previous DVT. There are a number of reasons for considering laparoscopic cholecystectomy patients to be at increased risk for developing DVT. First, the increased intra-abdominal pressure which accompanies adequate pneumoperitoneum impedes venous return to some extent, just as Valsalva manoeuvre does. Secondly, many surgeons prefer to place the patient in a reverse Trendelenburg position to obtain better exposure; this also leads to a relative venous stasis in the pelvis and lower extremities. Additionally, a number of these patients are obese, a condition known to predispose to DVT[32-5].

Equipment

Compared with open cholecystectomy, laparoscopic cholecystectomy requires an enormous amount of equipment, which may be grouped into three categories: video equipment, laparoscopic tools and energy sources.

Video equipment

One of the most significant advances in laparoscopic surgery occurred when the video camera was applied to the laparoscope. This marriage of two technologies opened the gateway to unprecedented possibilities in laparoscopic technique. For the first time, not only the surgeon but his entire team could visualize the peritoneal cavity concurrently. This allowed true 'informed' assistance by other members of the operative team. No longer would they have to guess what was occurring at the other end of the scope. This video technology is quite possibly the most important factor in the tremendous growth in laparoscopic surgery in recent years.

Elements of the system include:

- the telescope
- the light transmission cable
- the camera head
- the processing unit
- the auto-irising light source
- the high resolution video monitor(s).

Telescopes are available in a variety of sizes and optical configurations. Most popular sizes include the 10 mm and 5 mm diameter. A 0° wide angle is the most popular, but 30° scopes may be useful in certain circumstances, eg inspecting the porta hepatis from the umbilical port in a massively obese patient whose hepatic flexure of the colon would otherwise obscure the view with a 0° scope.

Older models of cameras relied on 'tube-type' image generation and were characterized by the rather bulky size of the unit which limited the manoeuvrability and attachment to the scope. With the development of 'chip' technology, 300 000 CCDs (controlled charge devices), could be packaged into a wafer-thin space approximately 1 cm². This obviously allowed production of much smaller cameras which would easily fit into the palm of one's hand, and which facilitated both attachment to, and movement of, the scope.

More sophisticated models incorporate three such chips in one head, thereby improving both colour and resolution. The chips generate an electrical signal which is sent to the processing unit where it is manipulated before being sent to the light source. From there it travels to the video monitor where it may be viewed.

The primary function of the light source is to generate a high-intensity beam which is transmitted to the telescope via an optic cable. Most current models use xenon as the source. Equally important as generation of the light, however, is control of its intensity. This is achieved by sophisticated models which incorporate an automatic iris function into the light source itself. Logistically, the intensity of the signal which is sent from the camera processor to the light source is 'read' by the auto-iris mechanism, and the output of the light source is either dimmed or enhanced depending on the incoming intensity.

This function becomes very important when the scope has to be moved alternately closer and farther from the object inside the peritoneal cavity on a routine basis. Without this function, the resultant image would be either too dark or too light half of the time. After the signal from the camera has been sent from the camera processor to the light source, it travels to the video monitor where it can be viewed by the operating team. It is essential for the video monitor(s) to have high resolution (more than 400 lines) capabilities, to allow the precise identification of anatomical structures needed for accurate dissection.

Laparoscopic instruments

Laparoscopic tools include those which are used to create and maintain a workspace in the abdominal cavity (pneumoperitoneum), those which are used to grasp, cut and dissect tissues, those which are used to ligate, clip or suture vessels and other structures, those which are used to maintain a clear field (suction and irrigation devices), and ancillary devices which facilitate completion of the procedure.

The Verres needle, with its spring-loaded safety tip, is most commonly used to establish pneumoperitoneum through a small incision at the umbilicus. Although the flow of gas (usually carbon dioxide) is somewhat limited through the needle, its safety makes it desirable as an initial 'blind' puncture device. Using flexible tubing, this needle is connected to an insufflator.

Today's insufflators are characterized by their ability to achieve high flow rates (typically 4–9 l/min) and to regulate the intra-abdominal pressure without exceeding a preset maximum limit. Insufflators which do not have capability to flow at 4 l or more per minute are usually not adequate in operative laparoscopy. Those which do not have automatic shut-off devices when a preset pressure limit is reached, are unsafe.

A variety of access ports are available. Both reusable and disposable devices may be used. The reusable units are less costly, but the disposable trocars are usually sharper and have a safety shield which helps protect the viscera. The surgeon should use the trocars and sleeves with which he is most comfortable, and which are the safest and most cost-effective for the patient.

Laparoscopic hand tools are proliferating rapidly. There are numerous grasping forceps, angled dissecting forceps, scissors, retractors and needle holders of differing styles. The surgeon must choose according to preference and what is available. For laparoscopic cholecystectomy, a basic set of instruments would include at least two grasping forceps to manipulate the gallbladder, one or more angled dissecting forceps, scissors, clip appliers, and extraction forceps to remove the gallbladder from the peritoneal cavity. Conventional instruments to close the fascia and skin should also be available.

Energy sources

These devices are used to perform functions which would be more time-consuming, difficult or even impossible with conventional mechanical laparoscopic equipment. Included in this category are heat-generating units such as endocoagulators, diathermy units and lasers. Newer energy sources are currently being developed; their application in laparoscopic surgery awaits further study.

Endocoagulators achieve their effect by heating tissue to obtain coagulation, necrosis or denaturation of protein. While they have been useful in gynaecological surgery for tubal interruption, their use in laparoscopic biliary tract surgery has been limited.

Diathermy units generate electrical currents which pass through tissue and also cause warming, protein denaturation, coagulation and necrosis, depending on the amount, type and duration of the current. These devices are available in either unipolar or bipolar modalities. Bipolar units are considered safer because the entire circuit within the patient exists between the electrodes at the tip of the hand-held instrument. Unipolar units have been criticized because the electrical circuit travels from the hand-held instrument, through the patient, to a grounding plate and to the generator. This arrangement theoretically threatens other organs which may accidentally be involved in this circuit, ie the accidental 'bowel burn' which can occur if exposed metal from a hand-held instrument passes too close to the intestine.

While much has been made of this potential risk in the gynaecological literature, recent experience in laparoscopic general surgery indicates that such risk may not be as great as once suspected[36,37]. Certainly, if a surgeon chooses to use this modality, he must take proper precautions to avoid inadvertent electrical injury to the patient.

Lasers represent the latest entry into the energy-source armamentarium. These devices generate a specific wavelength of light of extremely high intensity. The characteristics of this light – including collimation, coherence, and monochromaticity – enable lasers to have significant photobiothermal effects on tissue.

A variety of machines are available, each with its own special advantages and limitations. Each laser name is based on the medium which is used to produce its specific wavelength of light. For example, argon lasers house argon gas, which after excitation produces visible light in the 488–512 nm wavelength. Carbon dioxide lasers produce light in the far infrared portion of the electromagnetic spectrum at 10 600 nanometres, well outside the visible spectrum. Nd:YAG lasers use a crystal composed of yttrium, aluminium and garnet which is doped with neodymium as the laser medium. When this crystal is excited, it produces a wavelength of 1064 nanometres. If this wavelength is passed through a potassium titanyl phosphate (KTP) crystal, the wavelength is halved to 532 nm.

Obviously, there are numerous media available with which to construct lasers. A brief sample of lasers used in the medical/surgical arena includes:

- CO_2
- helium-neon
- KTP
- Nd:YAG
- Ho:YAG
- tuneable dye
- excimer.

Lasers are selected for use according to the specific tissue effects which each achieves. These effects are generally wavelength-specific. So, whereas carbon dioxide laser light is almost completely absorbed by tissue with high water content, that of argon, KTP and Nd:YAG is not. Similarly, while dark tissue highly absorbs all these wavelengths, light tissue does not absorb KTP and argon wavelengths to a significant degree. Nd:YAG lasers have tissue effects which depend not only on the 1064 nm wavelength, but also on the method of delivery of the light to the tissue. Free beam non-contact Nd:YAG light applied via a flexible fibreoptic bundle penetrates tissue much more deeply than the same light applied via a synthetic sapphire contact tip. Also, whereas non-contact Nd:YAG light penetrates lightly pigmented tissue rather poorly, the contact tip application penetrates effectively and precisely.

In general, most lasers are considerably more precise and cause much less adjacent tissue damage than electrical diathermy units currently in use. Certainly they present less of an electrical hazard, since no electrical current flows into the patient. The main risks are thermal burns to tissue which may encounter the free beam (for those lasers which use free beams). Ocular hazards are also a potential source of injury since most laser light is absorbed by some part of the human eye; so proper eye protection must be ensured.

With the recent surge of interest in operative laparoscopy for the general surgeon, came an intense interest in laser applications for these procedures. The benefits of electrical safety, high level of precision and minimal adjacent tissue damage seemed to make lasers ideal for laparoscopic surgery.

Unfortunately, there has been much confusion regarding the appropriate place for lasers in this revitalized field in the past few years. Proponents of laser use, often seemingly too closely aligned to particular manufacturers, not only rationalized their preference for the laser, but carried their arguments to the extreme by suggesting that the use of any other energy source was tantamount to malpractice. Advocates of electrosurgery, on the other hand, often suggested (without substantial evidence) that the use of the laser was all but irrational.

The dispute raged through most of 1990, with the true advantages and disadvantages of each modality often lost in the rhetoric. In fact, both modalities are very useful and each may be used very effectively to achieve a superb laparoscopic result. This author prefers to use a Nd:YAG contact tip laser to perform laparoscopic cholecystectomy, because of its precision, lack of adjacent tissue damage, lack of smoke generation, lack of visual distortion, its safety and its inherent tissue effects[38]. Others may prefer different energy sources for their work. These differences in preference should not be allowed to obscure the real essence of the discussion, which is how to perform laparoscopic cholecystectomy.

Operating theatre design

Since a large amount of equipment is required to perform video-enhanced laparoscopic surgery, the theatre must be big enough to house it comfortably without obstructing the surgeon, the anaesthetist or the nursing personnel. While the exact location of the equipment may vary, one suitable arrangement is shown in Figure 4.1. The operating table is centrally located. The anaesthetist and his equipment are located at the head of the table in the usual site. It is important for the anaesthetic equipment trolley to be placed far enough from the head of the table to allow for placement of the surgeon's video monitor trolley at, or cephalad to, the right shoulder. This allows the primary surgeon to have unobstructed viewing. The insufflator should be located on this cart, so that the surgeon may easily monitor the insufflation pressures throughout the case and be instantly aware of any alterations that might prove hazardous to the patient.

If a first assistant is employed, he stands on the patient's right side, opposite the surgeon. The scrub nurse is located to the assistant's right. Her instrument table may be located either behind them or at the foot of the table. If a camera operator is used, he is located to the left of the primary surgeon. The assistant's and scrub nurse's video monitor trolley is located opposite the other monitor, where both of them can see the screen.

Light sources, cameras and video-recording equipment may be placed on either trolley. The laser and the laser safety nurse are most commonly placed at the foot of the table, or behind and to the left of the primary surgeon. Ancillary devices such as suction and irrigation machines may be placed where the tubing path to the patient does not interfere with the movements of the operating team.

The room should be properly lit throughout the case. Some surgeons have developed the unusual and dangerous habit of turning off all lights in the room

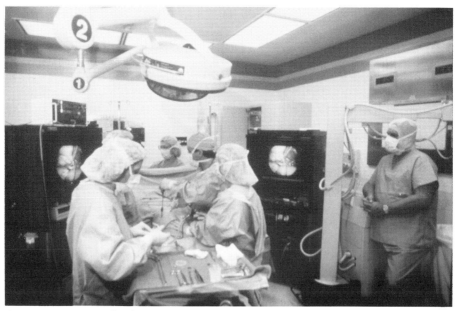

Figure 4.1: An example of operating theatre layout.

after the peritoneal cavity is entered with the scope. This is only mentioned to be condemned. This practice obviously increases the likelihood of accidents occurring during the case, such as wrong instrument selection or passage between the scrub nurse and the surgeon. If glare seems to be a problem on the monitor surface, the trolley should be oriented to minimize this effect. Only if absolutely necessary, should the room lights be dimmed slightly to allow better visualization of the monitors.

Some surgeons prefer to have an open laparotomy set immediately available for use in the event of laparoscopic catastrophe. There is certainly nothing wrong with this practice, although the necessity of such measures will probably decrease with experience. More importantly, however, the surgeon must be provided with an adequate amount of appropriate laparoscopic equipment! It is almost impossible to manage with substandard laparoscopic equipment.

Operative Technique

Overview

Laparoscopic cholecystectomy may be performed in a number of ways. It may be accomplished by employing as many as four people at the operating table, or as few as two. It may involve the use of diathermy or laser. It may require the use of sophisticated (and expensive) equipment or the use of seemingly mundane instruments in innovative ways. This presentation will emphasize the ability to perform with a single surgeon and a single scrub nurse. While mechanical devices are used to control some forceps and the camera, these instruments could just as easily be controlled by assistant surgeons or camera operators.

By featuring the single surgeon–single scrub nurse technique, it is hoped that the reader will begin to focus not only on the advantages of the new technology, but also on the ability to use such advanced equipment in the most efficient manner. After all, the surgeon's goal should not just be to apply newer techniques, but to use them prudently to improve patient outcome. Too often, surgeons rush to the latest technological advances without regard to the financial consequences of their activities. It would seem wise to incorporate these new ideas about gallbladder surgery into a rational programme that is least costly, most effective in treating the disease, and least injurious to the patient physically, emotionally and financially. Laparoscopic cholecystectomy is a procedure that is inherently well-suited to such application.

The conduct of the operation may be artificially divided into the following segments:

- patient preparation and positioning
- establishing the pneumoperitoneum
- primary port placement
- inserting the scope and accessing the video system
- inspection of the peritoneal cavity
- secondary port placement
- dissection of the triangle of Calot
- cholangiograms
- dissection of the gallbladder from the liver
- treatment of the operative site
- gallbladder extraction
- closure.

Each segment involves specific manoeuvres which facilitate its completion. Additionally, certain precautions taken in each of these areas will minimize the chances of surgical misadventure.

Patient preparation and positioning

Patients should be properly informed about the operation. It is useful, but not mandatory, for the patient to use a laxative or an enema on the day prior to surgery in order to reduce the amount of stool in the colon, which may on occasion cause difficulty in retraction of the hepatic flexure away from the liver. Preoperative shower with antibacterial soap decreases the chances of infectious problems. Smoking should be strongly discouraged or prohibited prior to surgery.

Antithrombotic prophylaxis, either with heparin or with pulsatile stockings, is used in all patients. Increased intra-abdominal pressure and the use of reverse Trendelenburg position predispose to venous stasis. Prophylactic antibiotics are used in all cases at this time; one dose is all that is required.

The patient is placed in a supine position on the operating table. After induction of general anaesthetic, a Foley urinary catheter and an orogastric tube are applied. The gastric tube is placed through the mouth in order to avoid nasal irritation. Its use to decompress the stomach is often essential to allow visualization of the porta hepatis. Additionally, decompression of the stomach is thought to decrease the amount of postoperative nausea experienced by the patient. It is removed when the case is completed. The patient is then prepared and draped in the usual fashion for abdominal surgery. Once the equipment tables and trolleys are in position, and all device cables and tubings are properly routed, the patient is ready for the operation.

Establishing the pneumoperitoneum

Pneumoperitoneum may be established by one of two methods: blind puncture or open laparoscopy[39]. In the blind puncture method, a spring-loaded Verres needle with a protective blunt tip is inserted through a small incision at the umbilicus. The incision may be made in a transverse or vertical direction depending on the patient's skin folds and on surgeon preference. The author prefers a vertical incision extending from the mid-point of the umbilicus to the 6 o'clock position. Surprisingly, this location provides little chance for infection, and the cosmetic effects are excellent. By making the incision *in* the umbilicus, the surgeon is entering the thinnest portion of the abdominal wall. This allows for much easier extraction of the gallbladder from this site later.

Before the needle is inserted, some surgeons prefer to place the patient in a slight 10°–15° Trendelenburg position, supposedly to allow the viscera to 'fall' cephalad and out of the path of the needle. This author questions whether such slight Trendelenburg really has much effect, and therefore prefers a neutral supine position.

Most importantly, the anterior abdominal wall must be elevated by the surgeon and/or his assistant while the needle is inserted. Some surgeons have advocated the use of towel clips on either side of the umbilicus as handles for this manoeuvre. This practice seems questionable, since with such action usually only the skin and subcutaneous tissue is elevated. It is crucial to elevate the entire thickness of the abdominal wall at the umbilicus, which can only be done effectively by grasping the abdominal wall with one's hand. If the entire thickness of the abdominal wall is not elevated, either the needle will be placed in an extraperitoneal anterior location, or inadvertent perforation of viscera or vessels will occur.

Some surgeons prefer to insert the needle in a caudad direction to avoid injury to the great vessels. Others insert it perpendicular to the abdominal wall, taking great care to limit the depth of penetration. This can be done either by placing the index finger alongside the shaft of the needle to a preselected level, or by actually holding the shaft of the needle between the thumb and index finger of the insertion hand at the same location. Confirmation of the intraperitoneal location of the needle tip may be made by a variety of methods including the saline drop test, the Palmer test, or by simply checking the intra-abdominal pressure on the insufflator;

the pressure should be very low (less than 4–6 mmHg) at this time. Once the placement is confirmed, the abdomen is insufflated until 'adequate' tympany is achieved. There is no absolute amount of carbon dioxide which must be instilled for 'adequate' distension to occur, but generally 2–4 l are required. The pressure should never exceed 15 mmHg, to prevent problems with venous return. After adequate distension is obtained, the Verres needle is removed.

The alternative method of accessing the peritoneal cavity through open laparoscopy involves the same type of incision at the umbilicus, although it is usually slightly larger. The fascia is incised under direct vision as well. The size of the wound should be as small as possible to allow a secure seal around the sheath after its placement. Prior to placement of the sheath, however, stay sutures are placed in the fascia on either side of the wound.

The specially designed cannula, with its blunt-tipped obturator and its external movable cone, is then inserted into the abdomen while gentle upward traction is placed on the stay sutures. Next the external cone is secured in position on the sheath and the stay sutures are secured to cleats on the sheath. These two manoeuvres have the effect of closing the fascia snugly up to the cone and external sheath to prevent leakage of carbon dioxide and loss of pneumoperitoneum. The insufflation tubing is attached to a hub on this sheath and the abdomen insufflated in the same manner as above. Although the stay sutures limit the mobility of the primary port, there is still adequate range of motion to allow performance of the operative procedure.

Primary port placement

A 10 mm port is usually required to allow insertion of the scope. Some surgeons use an 11 mm port here, but are then required to use a reducing sleeve to prevent leakage of carbon dioxide around the scope. This port is inserted through the same incision used for the Verres needle. The incision should be just large enough to accept the port, otherwise leakage of carbon dioxide or displacement of the sleeve will occur. Again, the anterior abdominal wall must be elevated manually to avoid injury to underlying viscera. It is important here to avoid orientation of the trocar in too caudad a direction.

Two problems may occur in this situation. If the trocar is angled too far inferiorly, it may terminate in the subcutaneous tissue or the preperitoneal space. Additionally, if it does reach the peritoneal cavity, it will be semi-permanently oriented towards the pelvis, causing great difficulty in viewing the upper abdomen. Obviously an orientation more perpendicular to the abdominal wall will provide greater range of movement of the scope. Certainly the risk of injury to underlying structures must be taken into account when using this method. However, certain precautions will make insertion safe. Placement of the index finger alongside the sheath as it is inserted will help limit the depth of penetration of the sharp trocar. Additionally, the use of disposable trocars with spring-loaded safety shields helps prevent injury to underlying structures.

Once the sheath is placed inside the preperitoneal cavity, the trocar is removed and the carbon dioxide tubing is connected to its hub on the port. The insufflator is then immediately checked to ensure that the pressure readings are appropriate. Attention is then directed to insertion of the scope.

Inserting the scope, accessing the video system and inspecting the abdomen

The laparoscope is prepared by attaching the light cable from the light source to the terminal near the eyepiece. The camera is attached to the eyepiece, and its other terminal is connected to the camera processing unit. If an optical filter is required (as with some lasers), it is interposed between the eyepiece and the camera.

The scope is then inserted into the preperitoneal cavity and the inspection is performed. Peritoneoscopy is performed prior to insertion of second-ary ports.

Secondary port placement

Appropriate placement of secondary ports is essential to the efficient con-duct of the operation. Although a variety of locations for these ports has been used, certain preferences have evolved (*see* Figure 4.2). Usually three secondary ports are placed in the right upper quadrant. Although the approximate location is shown on the surface diagram, the exact placement is determined by direct visualization of the peritoneal cavity. A 10 mm port is established in the epigastrium just to the right of the

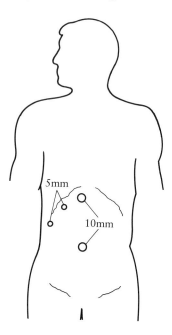

Figure 4.2: Secondary port placement.

falciform ligament approximately 3–4 cm inferior to the costal margin. A 5 mm port is placed directly over the fundus of the gallbladder as it rests in its undisturbed position; this port is located approximately in the mid-clavicular line 3 cm inferior to the costal margin; forceps introduced through it will be used to control the neck of the gallbladder. The final 5 mm port is placed in the anterior axillary line 3 cm inferior to the right costal margin; forceps introduced through it will be used to control the fundus of the gallbladder.

Once all ports have been established, grasping forceps are inserted through the two 5 mm sites. Forceps placed through the most lateral port are used to grasp the fundus of the gallbladder and displace it over the liver edge in a cephalad direction. It may be controlled either by a first assistant or by a mechanical device since it remains relatively fixed throughout the operation (*see* Figure 4.3). Forceps inserted through the mid-clavicular port are used to manipulate the neck of the gallbladder, and are controlled by the left hand of the primary surgeon. Instruments inserted through the medial epigastric port are used to perform the dissection.

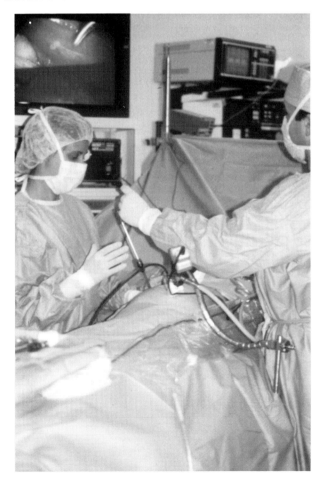

Figure 4.3: Grasp forceps in use.

Dissection of the triangle of Calot

One of the most potentially dangerous parts of the operation involves dissection in this area. The surgeon must remember that the anatomy will appear in an unfamiliar perspective. He must proceed very cautiously, identifying each structure in the triangle of Calot accurately prior to ligating or clipping or cutting the cystic artery and duct. Generally the safest approach involves starting the dissection as close to the gallbladder as possible and working toward the common duct. Curved forceps facilitate dissection in this area (*see* Figure 4.4). Scissors may be used to divide adhesions or peritoneum in this area. Once the artery is identified, it is secured with two or three titanium clips proximally and one or two clips distally. It may be divided now or later. The cystic duct is secured with two clips at the neck of the gallbladder. If no cholangiograms are performed, the duct is secured proximally with two or three clips, or with a ligature.

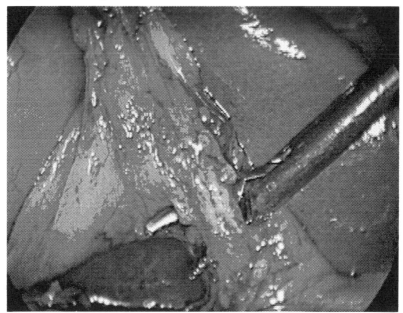

Figure 4.4: Curved forceps used in a dissection of the triangle of Calot.

Cholangiograms

The author strongly recommends performance of routine cholangiography for the following reasons: to establish proficiency, to define the anatomy and to evaluate the ductal system for disease. While the last reason may inspire debate, the first two reasons seem compelling enough to warrant this approach[40-9].

Two basic methods have been used to perform cholangiograms: the portal technique and the percutaneous technique. In 1989, Reddick and Olsen used the most lateral port to introduce a specially designed clamp which both placed and secured a cholangiogram catheter in the cystic duct. With this method, the remaining 5 mm grasping forceps must be repositioned to maintain exposure. Additionally, the radio-opaque clamp must be oriented so as not to obscure the ductal system on the film.

In 1990, Petelin developed the percutaneous technique for placement of the cholangiogram catheter[38]. In this method, a 14 French polyethylene sleeve is inserted through the abdominal wall in the cephalad direction, 2–3 cm medial to the mid-clavicular port. Through this sleeve the cholangiogram catheter is inserted into the peritoneal cavity where it is grasped by forceps inserted through the medial epigastric port. It is then placed into the cystic duct and secured into position with a clip placed across the catheter and duct. The clip is secured by the surgeon's right hand, while saline is injected through the catheter with his left hand. When there is enough resistance to injection, the clip application is stopped. This allows a water-tight seal at the insertion site and still enables sufficient flow for contrast injection into the ductal system. After completion of the films, the clip is easily removed and the catheter withdrawn from the duct.

The percutaneous method has several advantages over the portal method. Firstly, exposure is maintained since neither of the 5 mm grasping forceps needs to be moved. Secondly, no specialized clamp is required. Finally, the site of the partially applied clip is easily demonstrated on the films and therefore allows the surgeon precise delineation of the cystic duct–common duct junction.

Dissection of the gallbladder from the liver

After completion of the cholangiograms, the catheter is removed and the cystic duct is secured prior to its division. If the artery has not already been divided, it is divided now. Commonly, the posterior branch of the artery will also be encountered and will require clip application prior to its division.

Once this has been accomplished, the gallbladder may be dissected from the liver bed. To accomplish this with the laser, a suction–irrigation cannula is inserted through the medial epigastric port and the laser fibre is inserted through the centre of this cannula: thus it is possible to suck, irrigate and dissect conveniently all through the same port without having to insert and remove a variety of instruments. The precision afforded by the laser, and the magnification provided by the video system, allow an extremely precise dissection – accurate to within 1 mm. The lack of significant smoke production by the contact tip, and because the wavelength is outside the visible spectrum, ensure minimal disruption of the viewed image.

During the dissection it is important to keep gentle traction on the gallbladder to demonstrate the loose areolar plane that is present in all but the most inflamed cases. The surgeon accomplishes this just as in an open case, by manipulating the gallbladder with the forceps in his left hand. As more of the gallbladder wall is detached from the liver, it is helpful for the surgeon to reposition the mid-clavicular forceps closer to the line of dissection. This is referred to as the *reaching under* manoeuvre since the surgeon reaches under the body of the gallbladder to grasp the posterior wall and lift it off the liver.

This simple step provides significantly enhanced exposure for even the most intrahepatic gallbladder.

Treatment of the operative site

Once the gallbladder is completely detached from the liver, the most lateral forceps is removed and the gallbladder is placed above the liver where it is controlled by the mid-clavicular forceps.

Through the most lateral port a non-conductive fibreglass rod is inserted, to displace the liver in a cephalad direction and so allow inspection of the gallbladder bed. The deepest portion of this area may be exposed by using this same rod to displace the hepatic flexure of the colon and the duodenum inferiorly, while allowing the liver to 'float' freely. In almost every case this manoeuvre allows inspection of the previously placed clips and the cystic duct–common duct junction. Copious irrigation and suction may be used to remove any residual blood or debris from this area. When the surgeon is satisfied with the appearance of the operative site, the irrigation catheter and fibreglass rod are removed.

A 19 French fluted drain is then 'backloaded' through the medial epigastric port using an 8 mm introducer sleeve. Under direct vision on the monitor the drain is placed into the intra-abdominal portion of the most lateral port and advanced out onto the abdominal wall where it is clamped. The most lateral port is of course removed during this manoeuvre. The proximal portion of the drain is then placed in the gallbladder fossa with forceps introduced through the medial epigastric port. This drain is kept in place until the completion of the procedure.

After all ports have been removed and the abdomen has been decompressed, the drain is connected to suction while the other access sites are closed. This allows removal of any residual fluid and/or gas. If only minimal fluid has been discharged by the time the other sites have been closed, then the drain may be removed. If significant drainage is apparent, on the other hand, it may be left in place until the next day.

Gallbladder extraction

The most appropriate site for removal of the gallbladder is the umbilicus. Here the abdominal wall is the thinnest, and if extension of the incision is required it is better tolerated here than at any of the other sites.

In order to accomplish this, the scope must be moved to the medial epigastric port and the carbon dioxide tubing must be transferred to this site as well. The gallbladder is then transferred under direct vision on the monitor to forceps inserted through the umbilical port. This manoeuvre is facilitated if the surgeon holds the mid-clavicular forceps (with the gallbladder still attached) perpendicular to the abdominal wall with his left hand while he advances the umbilical forceps towards it, using the mid-clavicular forceps as a 'flagpole' to help guide the movements of his right-handed umbilical forceps.

Once the transfer has been accomplished, the gallbladder and the umbilical sheath are both withdrawn onto the abdominal wall. Usually only the neck of the gallbladder may protrude to the surface. Cautious gentle manipulation is required to deliver it further out of the peritoneal cavity. Occasionally, the gallbladder will need to be opened and decompressed at this time to allow its removal. Manual stone extraction may also be required. If both these manoeuvres fail to result in complete delivery, the fascia may be further incised as required. This is quite often the most appropriate decision, since it avoids disruption of the gallbladder or its loss back into the peritoneal cavity, both of which require considerable time and effort to correct.

Closure

After the gallbladder has been removed from the operative site, the fascia at the umbilicus is closed with a 0-Vicryl suture while the scope and the mid-clavicular port are still in place. The light from the scope illuminates the fascia at the umbilicus from its posterior aspect, and the minimal amount of carbon dioxide egress does not interfere significantly with visualization. The pneumoperitoneum reaccumulates once the fascia is closed adequately. The posterior aspect of the umbilicus may then be inspected to ensure that no excess tissue entrapment has occurred and that haemostasis is secure. Occasionally, a small amount of bleeding is identified at this time. It is easily controlled by introducing either the laser or a diathermy probe through the mid-clavicular port. A final inspection of the right upper quadrant is then made with the scope and the remaining ports are removed under direct vision.

The abdomen is then decompressed manually by the surgeon while the anaesthetist offers pronounced deep respiratory movements for the patient, thereby forcing the diaphragm inferiorly to remove any trapped suprahepatic gas or fluid. The fascia at the medial epigastric port and the skin at all sites are closed routinely. The drain is connected to suction while the remaining portal sites are closed. If minimal amounts of fluid are retrieved at this time, the drain is removed; otherwise it is connected to a suction device and left in place until the next day. Wounds are dressed with 1/2 inch steristrips as the only dressing.

Postoperative care

The orogastric tube and the Foley catheter are removed in the recovery room. Intravenous fluids are administered for approximately four hours after the patient leaves the recovery area. Patients are allowed to ingest liquids four hours after surgery and to advance to regular diet as tolerated; most patients tolerate a light meal within 12 hours of surgery. Mild nausea, which occasionally occurs, is usually relieved with conventional agents without the need for nasogastric decompression. A mild ileus is common. For this reason, a Dulcolax suppository is routinely administered within eight hours after completion of the operation. Although a low-grade temperature elevation is not uncommon, it rarely exceeds 99° F and usually requires no specific treatment. Patients are allowed out of bed as soon as they feel fit. Over 90% of patients are discharged from hospital within 24 hours. A significant number of patients may be safely discharged within four to six hours postoperatively.

Patients are advised to return for review within three or four days, after which they are normally discharged unless they have specific needs for prolonged care. They are allowed to return to their normal preoperative lifestyle and activities as their general well-being permits. Most are able to return to work within a week.

Conclusion

Laparoscopic cholecystectomy has proved to be an effective treatment for symptomatic gallbladder disease[50-5]. Over 95% of patients with gallbladder disease may be considered candidates for the procedure, and of this group more than 95% should be able to be completed laparoscopically. The procedure offers significant advantages over conventional open cholecystectomy, including less pain, less scarring, shorter hospitalization, less disruption of lifestyle and more rapid return to work. The procedure may be performed with a variety of energy sources, including diathermy and laser.

References

1   Dubois F, Icard P, Berthelot G and Levard H (1990) Coelioscopic cholecystectomy: Preliminary report of 36 cases. *Ann. Surg.* **211**: 60–2.

2   Reddick E, Olsen D, Daniell J, Saye W, McKernan B, Miller W and Hoback M (1989) Laparoscopic laser cholecystectomy. *Laser Med. Surg. News Adv.* **3**: 38–40.

3   Reddick E and Olsen D (1989) Laparoscopic laser cholecystectomy: a comparison with mini-lap cholecystectomy. *Surg. Endosc.* **3**: 131–3.

4   Dubois F, Berthelot G and Levard H (1991) Laparoscopic cholecystectomy: historic perspective and personal experience. *Surg. Lap. Endosc.* **1**: 52–7.

5   Reddick E, Baird D, Daniel J, Olsen D and Saye W (1990) Laparoscopic laser cholecystectomy. *Ann. Chir. Gyne.* **4**: 4–7.

6   Nahrwold D (1986) The biliary system. In: Sabiston DC (13th ed) *Textbook of surgery*. pp1128–37. WB Saunders, Philadelphia.

7   Hawasli A and Lloyd L (1991) Laparoscopic cholecystectomy the learning curve: Report of 50 patients. *Am. Surg.* **57**: 542–5.

8   Wolfe B, Gardiner B, Leary B, Frey C (1991) Endoscopic cholecystectomy: an analysis of complications. *Arch. Surg.* **126**: 1192–8.

9   Collet D, Magne E and Perissat J (1992) Laparoscopic cholecystectomy in the obese patient. *Surg. Endosc.* **6**: 186–8.

10 Aliperti G, Edmundowicz SA, Soper NJ and Ashley SW (1991) Combined endoscopic sphincterotomy and laparoscopic cholecystectomy in patients with choledocholithiasis and cholecystolithiasis. *Ann. Int. Med.* **115**: 783–5.

11 Cronin KJ, Kerlin MJ, Williams NN, Crowe J, MacMathuna P, Lennon J, Fitzpatrick JM and Gorey TF (1991) Endoscopic management of common duct stones with laparoscopic cholecystectomy. *I.J.M.S.* **160**: 265–7.

12 Cotton PB (1984) Endoscopic management of bile duct stones (apples and oranges). *Gut.* **25**: 587–97.

13 Carr-Locke DL (1990) Acute gallstone pancreatitis and endoscopic therapy. *Endosc.* **22**: 180–3.

14 Traverso L, Kozarek R, Ball T, Brandabur J, Hunter J, Jolly P, Patterson D, Ryan J, Thirlby R and Wechter D (1993) Endoscopic retrograde cholangopancreatography after laparoscopic cholecystectomy. *Am. J. Surg.* **165**: 581–6.

15 Petelin J (1991) Laparoscopic approach to common duct pathology. *Surg. Lap. Endosc.* **1**: 33–41.

16 Petelin J (1993) Laparoscopic approach to common duct pathology. *Am. J. Surg.* **165**: 487–91.

17 Hunter JG (1992) Laparoscopic transcystic common bile duct exploration. *Amer. J. Surg.* **163**: 53–8.

18 Scott-Coombes D and Thompson JN (1991) Bile duct stones and laparoscopic cholecystectomy. *Brit. Med. J.* **303**: 1281–2.

19 Fletcher DR (1991) Percutaneous (laparoscopic) cholecystectomy and exploration of the common bile duct: the common bile duct stone reclaimed for the surgeon. *Aust. NZ. J. Surg.* **61**: 814–15.

20 Arregui ME, Davis CJ, Arkush AM and Nagan RF (1992) Laparoscopic cholecystectomy combined with endoscopic sphincterotomy and stone extraction or laparoscopic choledocholscopy and electrohydraulic lithotripsy for management of cholelithiasis with choledocholithiasis. *Surg. Endosc.* **6**: 10–15.

21 Dion YM, Morin J, Dionne G and Dejoie C (1992) Laparoscopic cholecystectomy and choledocholithiasis. *C.J.S.* **35**: 67–74.

22 Shapiro SJ and Grundest W (1991) Laparoscopic exploration of the common bile duct: experience in 16 selected patients. *J. Laparoendosc. Surg.* **1**: 333–41.

23 Carroll BJ, Phillips EH, Daykhovsky L, Grundfest WS, Gershman A, Fallas M and Chandra M (1992) Laparoscopic choledochoscopy: an effective approach to the common duct. *J. Laparoendosc. Surg.* **2**: 15–21.

24   McAlhany JC and Sim R (1991) Laparoscopic exploration of the common duct with stone extraction. *J. S. Carolina Med. Assoc.* 375–7.

25   Smith P, Clayman RV and Soper NJ (1992) Laparoscopic cholecystectomy and choledochoscopy for the treatment of cholelithiasis and choledocholithiasis. *Surg.* **111**: 230–3.

26   Stoker ME, Leveillee RJ, McCann JC and Maini BS (1991) Laparoscopic common bile duct exploration. *J. Laparoendosc. Surg.* **1**: 287–93.

27   Sackier JM, Berci G and Paz-Partlow M (1991) Laparoscopic transcystic choledochotomy as an adjunct to laparoscopic cholecystectomy. *Amer. Surg.* **57**: 323–6.

28   Jacobs M, Verdeja JC and Goldstein HS (1992) Laparoscopic choledocho-lithotomy. *J. Laparoendosc. Surg.* **1**: 79–82.

29   DePaula A, Hashiba K, Bafutto M, Zago R and Machado M (1993) Laparoscopic antegrade sphincterotomy. *Surg. Laparoscop. Endosc.* **3**: 157–60.

30   Weber A, Bloom G, Allan T and Curry S (1991) Laparoscopic cholecystectomy during pregnancy. *Obstet. Gynec.* **78**: 58–9.

31   Soper N, Hunter J and Petrie R (1992) Laparoscopic cholecystectomy during pregnancy. *Surg. Endosc.* **6**: 115–17.

32   Moosa A, Lavelle-Jones M and Scott M (1986) Surgical complications. In: Sabiston DC (13th ed.) pp331–45 *Textbook of surgery*. WB Saunders, Philadelphia.

33   Bell W and Zuidema G (1979) Low dose heparin: Concern and perspectives. *Surg.* **85**: 469.

34   Flanc C, Kakkar V and Clarke M (1969) Postoperative deep vein thrombosis: Effect and intensive prophylaxis. *Lancet.* **1**: 477.

35   Kakkar V, Corrigan T and Fossard D (1975) International multicentre trial. Prevention of fatal postoperative embolism by low doses of heparin. *Lancet.* **2**: 45.

36   Hunter J (1993) Exposure, dissection and laser versus electrosurgery in laparoscopic cholecystectomy. *Amer. J. Surg.* **165**: 492–6.

37   Voyles C (1993) The laparoscopic buck stops here. *Amer. J. Surg.* **165**: 472–3.

38   Petelin J (1990) The argument for contact laser laparoscopic cholecystectomy. *Clin. Laser Monthly.* 71–4.

39   Fitzgibbons R, Annibali R and Litke B (1993) Gallbladder and gallstone removal, open versus closed laparoscopy and pneumoperitoneum. *Amer. J. Surg.* **165**: 497–504.

40   Hunter J (1991) Avoidance of bile duct injury laparoscopic cholecystectomy. *Amer. J. Surg.* **162**: 71–6.

41 Phillips E, Berci G, Carroll B, Daykhovsky L, Sackier J and Paz-Partlow M (1990) The importance of intraoperative cholangiography during laparoscopic cholecystectomy. *Amer. Surg.* **56**: 792–5.

42 Handy J, Rose S, Nieves A, Johnson R, Hunter J and Miller F (1991) Intraoperative cholangiography: use of portable fluoroscopy and transmitted images. *Radiol.* **181**: 205–7.

43 Blatner M, Wittgen C, Andrus C and Kaminiski D (1991) Cystic duct cholangiography during laparoscopic cholecystectomy. *Arch. Surg.* **126**: 646–9.

44 Pietrafitta J, Schultz L, Graber J, Josephs L and Hickok D (1991) Cholecystcholangiography during laparoscopic cholecystectomy: Cholecystcholangiography or cystic duct cholangiography. *J. Laparoendosc. Surg.* **1**: 197–206.

45 Sackier J, Berci G, Phillips E, Carroll B, Shapiro S and Paz-Partlow M (1991) The role of cholangiography in laparoscopic cholecystectomy. *Arch. Surg.* **126**: 1021–6.

46 Gompertz R, Rhodes M and Lennard T (1992) Laparoscopic cholangiography: An effective and inexpensive technique. *Br. J. Surg.* **79**: 23–4.

47 Cantwell D (1992) Routine cholangiography during laparoscopic cholecystectomy. *Arch. Surg.* **127**: 483–4.

48 Lillemoe K, Yeo C, Talamini M, Wang B, Pitt H and Gadacz T (1992) Selective cholangiography: current role in laparoscopic cholecystectomy. *Ann. Surg.* **215**: 669–76.

49 Mirizzi P (1936) Operative cholangiography. *S. G. O.* **64**:702–10.

50 Airan M, Appel M and Berci G *et al.*, (1992) Retrospective and prospective multi-institutional laparoscopic cholecystectomy study organized by the Society of American Gastrointestinal Endoscopic Surgeons. *Surg. Endosc.* **6**: 169–76.

51 Spaw A, Reddick E and Olsen D (1991) Laparoscopic laser cholecystectomy: analysis of 500 procedures. *Surg. Laparosc. Endosc.* **1**: 2–7.

52 Zucker K, Flowers J, Bailey R, Graham S, Buell J and Imbembo A (1993) Laparoscopic management of acute cholecystitis. *Amer. J. Surg.* **165**: 508–14.

53 Gadacz T (1993) US experience with laparoscopic cholecystectomy. *Amer. J. Surg.* **165**: 450–4.

54 Gollan J *et al.*, (1992) National Institutes of Health Consensus Development Conference Statement: gallstones and laparoscopic cholecystectomy September 14–16, 1992. *J. Laparoendosc. Surg.* **3**: 77–90.

55 Meyers W *et al.*, (1991) The Southern Surgeons Club: a prospective analysis of 1518 laparoscopic cholecystectomies. *New Eng. J. Med.* **324**: 1073–8.

5

Laparoscopic Appendicectomy

HUBA BAJUSZ AND MICHAEL J. McMAHON

Historical perspective

Appendicectomy is one of the most common abdominal operations. It is usually performed using a small incision in the right iliac fossa, but as every surgical resident comes to appreciate, the traditional gridiron incision has a number of disadvantages. Location of the appendix can be difficult when the organ lies in an ectopic position such as deep in the pelvis, high under the liver or behind the caecum. Abdominal exploration through a gridiron incision is limited to the region of the right iliac fossa, and the diagnosis often remains uncertain if the appendix itself is normal. Complete peritoneal lavage is often difficult with patients with generalized peritonitis and finally, as in any laparotomy, appendicectomy can be a source of complications such as:

- infection or herniation of the wound

- abscess

- intestinal obstruction due to adhesions

- chronic wound pain.

Later complications include:

- bowel obstruction

- infertility in females

- chronic lower abdominal pain.

Laparoscopic appendicectomy appears to offer the potential to reduce the frequency of complications of classic appendicectomy and to facilitate more precise diagnosis.

The first laparoscopically guided appendicectomy appears to have been performed by De Kok[1] in 1977. He removed the appendix via a mini-laparotomy after confirming the diagnosis and the position of the organ laparoscopically. Complete laparoscopic appendicectomy was first performed in 1983 by the German gynaecologist Semm[2], who recommended that the technique should be reserved for the uninflamed appendix only.

Laparoscopically directed and assisted surgery for the acutely inflamed appendix was reported in 1985 by Flemming[3] from New South Wales, and in 1986 by Wilson[4] from Sydney. In 1987, Schreiber in Germany[5] reported laparoscopic appendicectomy for the treatment of acute appendicitis, and since then several further reports have appeared[6–8] including large numbers of patients treated routinely by the laparoscopic approach[9–12].

Pier *et al.*[11] reported 625 successful laparoscopic operations of which only 14 (2%) were converted to an open procedure because of operative complications such as bleeding or dense adhesions. Acute inflammation was confirmed by histology in 71% of the patients. Seventy (of the 625 patients) had 'phlegmonous' appendicitis; the appendix was gangrenous in only ten patients, and perforated in only nine. The low incidence of gangrenous or perforated appendix suggests that there was a low threshold for operative intervention. Chronic inflammation was found in 15% of cases and a normal appendix was removed in less than 14%. Three patients developed postoperative abscess with paralytic ileus and required laparotomy, and 14 patients developed cellulitis around the umbilical puncture site, which was successfully treated with antibiotics alone in each instance.

Instrumentation required for laparoscopic appendicectomy

The following instruments are adequate for routine laparoscopic appendicectomy:

- Verres needle

- 10 mm and 5 mm laparoscopes (0° or 30°)

- operating trocars and cannulae (2 x 10 mm, 2 x 5.5 mm)

- blunt dissecting forceps

- curved dissecting forceps

- scissors

- Babcock forceps

- catgut ligature loops and applier

- diathermy blade or hook

- diathermy forceps

- suction–irrigation cannula

- clip applicator device

- 10–5 mm reducing sleeve

- bag or pouch for the mobilized appendix

- high-flow insufflator, high-definition video camera and high-output light source.

Additional instruments, such as retractors, needle-holders etc may be required for complicated cases.

Basic operative technique

Laparoscopic appendicectomy requires general anaesthesia with endotracheal intubation and full abdominal wall relaxation. The patient is asked to void urine prior to the operation, and a urethral catheter is only used if the bladder is found to be enlarged by palpation, or on inspection with the laparoscope. The stomach is decompressed with a nasogastric tube. One dose of an iv broad-spectrum antibiotic or of metronidazole is given routinely at the introduction of the general anaesthetic, and the decision to give more than one dose of antibiotic is made at operation if there is free pus or extensive peritoneal contamination.

The patient is placed supine on the operating table. All skin incision sites are infiltrated with bupivacaine (0.5% with 1:100,000 adrenaline) to minimize postoperative pain. The operation commences with a 1 cm curved, infra-umbilical incision. The abdominal wall is elevated infra-umbilically with one hand and the Verres needle is placed straight into the peritoneal cavity angled towards the right side of the pelvis so that the capnoperitoneum can be established. The operator gradually employs a pressure limit of 12 mmHg – lower pressure if possible. A 10 mm disposable trocar and cannula is inserted into the abdominal cavity through the infra-umbilical incision and angled towards the right iliac fossa. During diagnostic visualization of the peritoneal cavity with a 10 mm laparoscope, or at other stages of the operation, the operating table may be tilted in different directions to provide optimal access. This is especially valuable in an obese patient or when there are distended bowel loops.

In a patient with a pre-existing midline abdominal scar it is safer to start by insertion of the Verres needle and the initial cannula in the right sub-costal area (see below) or by using the Hasson method[13], which is an open mini-laparotomy at the umbilicus to access the peritoneal cavity.

Routinely, the second cannula (5.5 mm) is inserted 2 cm superior to the pubic symphysis in the midline (see Figure 5.1). A reusable trocar and cannula are quite suitable because they can be introduced under direct vision. Trauma to the bladder is avoided by direct inspection, and by catheterization if an enlarged bladder is present. Initial diagnostic laparoscopy is performed using blunt forceps to manipulate intra-abdominal organs. The small bowel is inspected for the presence of a Meckel's diverticulum if there is no evidence of appendicitis. In female patients, the ovaries, Fallopian tubes and uterus are routinely inspected. Thorough inspection of the intra-abdominal organs often requires the insertion of a third cannulation site. If it is needed, or if the decision is made to remove the appendix, a third 5 mm cannula is inserted quite low (especially in young women or girls) in the right iliac fossa to grasp the appendix. The exact position of this cannula depends upon the position of the appendix. If only a 10 mm laparoscope is available, the suprapubic cannula will also need to be 10 mm.

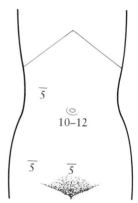

Figure 5.1: Basic operative technique: the second cannula is inserted superior to the pubic symphysis in the midline.

It is often necessary to divide adhesions using electrocautery or scissors before the appendix can be approached. 'Fresh' adhesions are usually divided easily with a sweeping action of blunt or curved dissecting forceps. The tip of the appendix may be visible, but most usually it is in a concealed position and the base of the appendix is first visualized by retracting the caecal pole in a cephalad direction by grasping the anterior taenium with forceps. It is sometimes helpful to insert an additional 5 mm cannula in the mid-clavicular line just below the right costal margin in order to pull the caecal pole in a cephalad direction so that the appendix base is raised up and can be grasped or mobilized.

Once the base of the appendix has been visualized, it is usually easy to mobilize it completely by sweeping away adhesions with a pair of blunt forceps. Difficulty may be caused by impairment of vision from adjacent dilated loops of small bowel and omentum, and under these circumstances, if tilting the table is insufficient to obtain good views, an additional 5 mm cannula on the left side of the abdomen enables viscera to be held down and out of the field of view with a triangular retractor such as the Endoflex (Electa Instruments Inc., Atlanta, GA, USA).

Mobilization of the appendix may be difficult if adhesions are mature and fibrous. An effective approach is to be patient and to combine careful blunt and occasional sharp dissection whilst the visible parts of the appendix are grasped firmly with Babcock forceps. The appendix tip can be grasped by various techniques. If thin (and relatively normal), it can be held in a pair of forceps introduced through the cannulation site in the right iliac fossa. If the appendix tip is inflamed and swollen, or gangrenous and friable, regular grasping forceps may be less satisfactory and toothed forceps will tend to tear the tissues. An alternative is to catch the appendix tip in a self-tightening catgut loop (Endoloop, Ethicon Ltd, Edinburgh, UK), which is then trimmed to leave a short 'tail' of catgut which can be grasped with forceps. The catgut may be left long and brought outside the abdomen in the manner of a stay suture using a suture retrieval device (Endoclaw, Surgical Innovations UK Ltd, Leeds, UK) which has the potential to leave all the cannulation sites free for instruments.

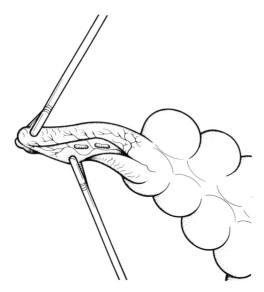

Figure 5.2: The appendix mesentery opens out like a fan.

Once the appendix has been mobilized, the tip is grasped so that the appendix mesentery is opened out like a fan (*see* Figure 5.2). A diathermy blade, blunt forceps or scissors are used to fashion 'windows' between the vessels of the meso-appendix. The 10 mm laparoscope is withdrawn and replaced by a 5 mm laparoscope inserted through the suprapubic cannulation site so that a clip applicator can be used through the umbilical site to ligate the mesenteric vessels with steel or titanium clips. The vessels and the meso-appendix are divided step by step until the base of the appendix has been fully mobilized (*see* Figure 5.3). Division of the meso-appendix close to the wall of the appendix makes haemostasis easier and, because the bulk of the resected appendix is kept to a minimum, it is more easily removed through the 10 mm umbilical cannulation site. Three chromic catgut ligatures (Endoloops) are placed around the appendix, siting the first directly at its caecal end, the second about 2–3 mm more distally and the third about 1 cm distal to the second (*see* Figure 5.4). The appendix is divided with either scissors or diathermy between the second and third ligatures. It is important that the appendix stump is secured carefully and safely (*see* Figure 5.5). The stump can be inverted as originally described by Semm[1] but it is usually not considered necessary to do so. In conventional surgery prospective, randomized studies have shown no advantages of inversion over simple ligation[14].

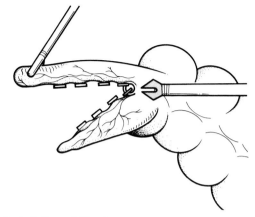

Figure 5.3: The base of the appendix is fully mobilized.

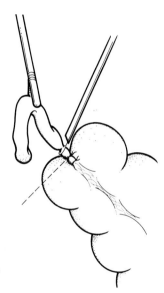

Figure 5.4: Three chromic catgut ligatures (Endo-loops) are placed around the appendix.

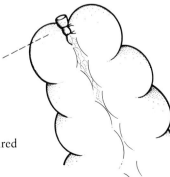

Figure 5.5: The appendix stump should be secured carefully and safely.

Finally, the appendix is pulled into a reduction sleeve introduced via the 10 mm cannula and removed together with the reduction sleeve, thereby preventing the contaminated tissue coming into contact with the abdominal wall or the cannula itself. If the appendix is too bulky for removal through the sleeve, it can be placed in a small bag (BERT, Scimed Ltd, Leeds, UK) and removed when the umbilical cannulation site has been converted to 20–25 mm diameter using a large cannula (it is unusual for this to be necessary). After removal of the appendix, the stump and mesentery are carefully examined to ensure that there is no bleeding and that the appendix stump is firmly closed. The region of the appendix, and a wider area if necessary, is then washed out with warm saline. We close the umbilical fascia with a size 1 polydioxone monofilament suture on a strong 'J'-shaped needle (Ethicon) and the skin with simple 3/0 nylon sutures. Adhesive plastic dressings are placed over each incision.

In our hands, the operating time has been between 25 and 55 minutes.

Postoperative care

The nasogastric tube is removed at the end of the procedure unless there is clinical ileus, and patients are encouraged to take diet *ad libitium*. Continued use of iv fluids and a nasogastric tube may be necessary in the toxic patients with perforated appendices. Patients may shower or bathe after surgery, the wounds being protected by the adhesive dressing. The pain after laparoscopic surgery is easily controlled in most patients with a mild oral analgesic such as paracetamol. Sutures are removed in five to seven days and the patient is usually reviewed once in the out-patient department about four weeks after the operation.

Alternative methods

Retrograde appendicectomy

In acutely inflamed cases the appendix may be too inflamed and friable for traction to be used. The most proximal part of the appendix is usually less necrotic and it may be easier to identify and create an opening in the appendix mesentery adjacent to the caecum prior to mobilization of the whole organ. The appendix can be then divided using ligatures tied internally or externally, or much more easily, although more expensively, using a combined stapler and knife (EndoGIA, US Surgical Corporation, Norwalk, CT, USA) — (*see* Figure 5.6). The appendix can then be removed retrogradely. If it is very friable this may be piecemeal, and it is important that all fragments are retrieved.

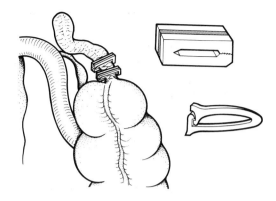

Figure 5.6: Division of the appendix using a combined stapler and knife.

Laparoscopically assisted appendicectomy

This technique is suggested only in patients with a thin abdominal wall, and a mobile caecum and appendix. It is probably more applicable to children than to adults. After the mesentery of the appendix has been divided, it is pulled through a 10 mm cannulation site placed directly over the caecum. Ligation, resection and disinfection of the appendix stump are performed outside the abdomen (*see* Figure 5.7). The appendix stump is then returned to the abdomen.

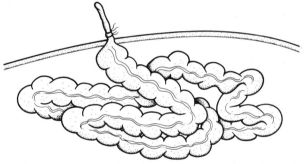

Figure 5.7: Ligation, resection and disinfection of the appendix stump are performed outside the abdomen.

Closure of the stump

The most frequently used method for closure of the appendix stump is the application of ligatures as pre-tied, sliding, Roeder loops (Endoloop). Alternatively, the stump may be ligated using either intra or extra abdominal knot tying techniques. Both locking absorbable clips and plastic-metal clips have been used to secure the stump. (Such clips have been used for many years to ligate the Fallopian tube.) A recently developed stapling device (EndoGIA) has been used for the division of the meso-appendix as well as closure of the appendix stump. The use of this device makes the operation quicker, but it needs a 12 mm operating cannula to introduce the stapling device and the technique is relatively expensive.

Alternative dissection techniques

Although it is usual to employ forceps or diathermy to dissect the appendix mesentery, other alternatives are available. The mesentery may be secured *en masse* using a linear stapler (EndoGIA). Dissection can be carried out with a contact Nd:YAG laser or a harmonic scalpel, but the advantages of these techniques remain to be established. Ligatures and sutures may be used as alternatives to staples for control of the mesentery of the appendix, but they are more time-consuming.

Problems during appendicectomy

The appendix is found to be normal

If the appendix is found to be normal, then other causes of abdominal pain must be sought. Free peritoneal fluid may give a clue to the correct diagnosis. Mesenteric adenitis may be associated with clear yellow free peritoneal fluid and enlarged mesenteric lymph nodes may be visualized. Perforation of a peptic ulcer is associated with bile-stained fluid, pus or recognizable food debris. Methylene blue can be introduced into the stomach through a nasogastric tube and may help to identify a perforation, but the fibrinous exudate and oedematous, inflamed tissues in the right upper quadrant are usually obvious. Duodenal perforation can be treated laparoscopically[15]. Faecal contents in the peritoneal cavity suggests colonic perforation, blood-stained fluid is characteristic of bowel infarction, and free blood suggests rupture of an aortic aneurysm or an ectopic pregnancy. After suction and lavage the source of the bleeding may be visualized, but if there is a large amount of blood and clot, conversion to laparotomy should be undertaken immediately.

If no other pathology is immediately apparent, a systematic laparoscopic examination should be performed in order to visualize the stomach, duodenum, gallbladder, and in women, the ovaries, Fallopian tubes and the uterus. The small bowel must be inspected for the presence of a Meckel's diverticulum or terminal ileitis, and the large bowel examined to exclude diverticulitis or tumour. Treatment (laparoscopic or conventional) can be decided when the diagnosis becomes apparent. Potentially, diagnostic laparoscopy can avoid up to 75% of 'unnecessary' appendicectomies[16-20] but it is still unclear whether appendicectomy should be carried out if a normal appendix is visualized and no other cause of symptoms is found. Whilst the argument used to justify routine removal of the appendix is used probably applies equally to the laparoscopic approach as to a conventional gridiron incision, it is probable that the appendix which is not overtly inflamed, but is the case of pain, will settle rapidly if left *in situ*. The consensus appears to favour a policy that the appendix should not be removed if it looks normal.

Retrocoecal position of the appendix

If the appendix is not visible because it occupies a retrocoecal position, the caecum may be mobilized by incising the peritoneum lateral to it with scissors or diathermy (just as at conventional surgery). Occasionally an additional 5 mm cannula may be needed to retract the ascending colon in order to put the peritoneum lateral to it 'on the stretch'.

Perforated appendix

Perforation is not an indication for conversion to an open appendicectomy, as long as the appendix can be mobilized. Care should be used when manipulating an oedematous or inflamed caecal wall. Fresh adhesions and a bulky and inflamed meso-appendix may bleed readily, but with patience and meticulous haemostasis the problems are soluble. Careful abdominal lavage should be carried out after removal of a perforated appendix so that all traces of pus are aspirated from the abdomen and pelvis.

Mickel's diverticulum

It is not usually possible to distinguish the clinical features of inflammation of a Meckel's diverticulum from those of acute appendicitis. A Meckel's diverticulum should be sought routinely if the appendix is found to appear normal. A diverticulum discovered incidentally need not be removed as routine, but laparoscopic diverticulectomy can be performed in a similar way to appendicectomy, if necessary, using the EndoGIA stapler if the mouth of the diverticulum is wide (*see* Figure 5.8). The small bowel can be examined by 'walking' atraumatic grasping forceps up the bowel from the ileocaecal valve.

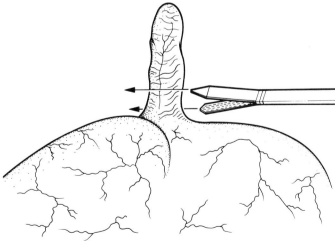

Figure 5.8: Laparoscopic diverticulectomy using the EndoGIA stapler.

Bleeding

Although bleeding is a potentially serious complication of laparoscopic appendicectomy it can be managed safely in most patients. Diathermy forceps, pre-tied Roeder loops, sutures and clips are generally used to control bleeding, and it is important for every laparoscopic surgeon to have had experience of these techniques using a simulator or trainer. Care should be taken to identify the precise source of the bleeding and the 'blind' application of clips or mass diathermy is to be condemned. If necessary, pressure from a pledgelet or swab can be used to gain control in the first instance. An efficient suction–irrigation system is important for safe control of bleeding.

Conversion to open operation

In the initial phase of laparoscopic work the interests of safety may dictate a low threshold for conversion to laparotomy. With experience the frequency of conversion falls. However, it is important to have a set of 'open' instruments in the operating theatre for immediate conversion if complications occur. Major bleeding does not allow the surgeon much time to convert to laparotomy.

Laparoscopy in elderly patients

The 'classical picture' of appendicitis may be attenuated in elderly patients. Pain is a less prominent feature. The more rapid course of appendicitis and delay in diagnosis more commonly results in gangrene and perforation. Laparoscopy early in the course of atypical cases may help to avoid delay in this group of patients. Elderly patients with cardiorespiratory problems may be at some risk of cardiac complications during abdominal insufflation. The main factor responsible is the increased intra-abdominal, and hence intrathoracic, pressure. This directly influences venous return and can cause reduction in cardiac output as well as increased intra-alveolar pressure[21]. These effects are well-compensated in patients with normal cardiopulmonary status, but less well-tolerated in elderly patients with chronic cardiopulmonary problems[22]. Patients with previously diagnosed cardiac or pulmonary disease need to be scrupulously monitored intraoperatively. The minimum pressure of carbon dioxide compatible with safe surgery should be used, and the patient's legs should be enclosed in elastic support stockings.

Laparoscopic appendicectomy in children

Valla *et al.*[12] reported collected data on 465 laparoscopic appendicectomies in children, with excellent results. There was a 3% incidence of minor postoperative complications and only 1.3% of the patients were converted to, or subsequently needed, laparotomy. In children it is relatively easy to perform the laparoscopically assisted operation, and this may be the most expedient technique when the child is small and only 'adult' laparoscopic instruments are available. The principal problem in the child is the small size of the abdomen, and the limited space which is available to the laparoscopic surgeon, but specialized paediatric instruments are being developed to help overcome these difficulties.

Laparoscopic appendicectomy in pregnancy

The diagnosis of acute appendicitis in pregnancy can be very difficult. There is a higher frequency of false diagnosis and there is a high rate of abortion and premature birth associated with advanced appendicitis. Diagnostic laparoscopy has been performed in many gynaecological centres on women of childbearing years suspected of having appendicitis. Recently, Schreiber[23] reported a series of laparoscopic appendicectomies in pregnancy without any complications. The size of the uterus is obviously of great importance. The position of the trocar insertion is modified according to the period of gestation, but after the 30th week of gestation there is certainly limited space for this kind of surgery (*see* Figures 5.9 and 5.10).

One theoretical argument against laparoscopic surgery in pregnancy is the fear of interference with the blood supply of the uterus by increased intra-abdominal pressure. However, an intra-abdominal pressure of 10–14 mmHg does not appear to cause significant risks[23].

It is often easier to decide to perform laparoscopy (diagnostic or surgical) in the pregnant woman than to intervene by laparotomy because of the less invasive nature of the procedure. Early intervention may prevent perforation of the appendix and decrease the risk of abortion. An additional potential advantage of the laparoscopic approach during pregnancy is a decreased incidence of incisional herniation[5]. Pregnancy, therefore, should not be considered a contraindication to laparoscopic surgery, as has been suggested by some authors[24], except in the third trimester.

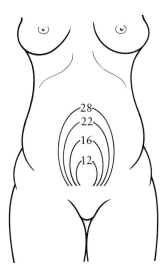

Figure 5.9: The position of the trocar insertion is modified according to the period of gestation.

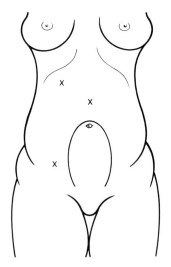

Figure 5.10: The position of the trocar insertion is modified according to the period of gestation.

Contraindications to laparoscopic appendicectomy

These include:

- end term pregnancy (third trimester)

- diffuse peritonitis with fibrinous plaques

- multiple previous abdominal operations

- known abdominal malignancy

- severe bleeding disorders (not an absolute contraindication, but be prepared to 'convert')

- inability to tolerate general anaesthesia.

Clinical results of laparoscopic appendicectomy

There are two reports of sufficient numbers of patients, with a clinical diagnosis of acute appendicitis submitted to laparoscopic appendicectomy, for an appraisal of success rate and complications to be assessed. In Germany, Pier et al.[11] reported 625 laparoscopic operations in 639 patients. The age range was 2–86 years. The usual reason for failure to carry out a laparoscopic procedure was unfamiliarity of the surgeon with the laparoscopic operation or unwillingness of the patient to undergo it. Appendicectomy was carried out in all cases, and there was evidence of acute inflammation in 70% of the removed appendices. It was necessary to convert only 14 operations to laparotomy (2%) and most conversions were during the author's initial experience. The complication rate was not reported, but subsequent laparotomy was needed to treat an abscess in two patients (both had perforated appendicitis) and paralytic ileus in another.

Laparoscopic appendicectomy in 465 children (3–16 years) was reported by Valla *et al.* from four centres in France[12]. The study combined 40 laparoscopic procedures with laparoscopic assisted operations. Conversion to laparotomy was necessary in five patients (1%). There were 17 intraoperative 'accidents' which included two visceral punctures, and 14 postoperative complications (3%). The latter included two hernias, three intraperitoneal abscesses, one fistula in a patient with Crohn's disease and two patients with intestinal obstruction (neither of whom needed laparotomy). Only 1.3% of the patients required a repeat operation.

These data suggest that laparoscopic appendicectomy is safe, widely applicable and associated with complication rates which are as low, or lower, than the conventional procedure. Only further experience, preferably in the setting of randomized trials, and using junior surgeons (who actually carry out appendicectomy) will enable a judgement of the precise advantages of the laparoscopic approach to be made.

References

1   De Kok H (1977) A new technique for resecting the non-inflamed knot-adhesive appendix through a mini-laparotomy with the aid of the laparoscope. *Arch. Chir. Neerl.* **29**:195–7.

2   Semm K (1983) Endoscopic appendectomy. *Endoscopy.* **15**:59–64.

3   Fleming JS (1985) Laparoscopically directed appendectomy. *Austr. N.Z. Obstet. Gynecol.* **25**:238–40.

4   Wilson T (1986) Laparoscopically assisted appendectomies. *Med. J. Aust.* **145**:551.

5   Schreiber JH (1987) Early experience with laparoscopic appendectomy in women. *Surg. Endosc.* **1**:211–16.

6   Gangal HT (1987) Laparoscopic appendectomy. *Endoscopy.* **19**:127–9.

7   Götz F, Pier A and Bacher C (1990) Modified laparoscopic appendectomy in surgery. *Surg. Endosc.* **4**:6–9.

8   Leahy PF (1989) Technique of laparoscopic appendectomy. *Br. J. Surg.* **76**:616.

9   Nowzaradan Y, Westmoreland J and McCarver CT (1991) Laparoscopic appendectomy for acute appendicitis. Indication and current use. *J. Laparoendosc. Surg.* **1**:247–57.

10 Patterson-Brown S, Thompson JN and Eckersley JR (1988) Which patient with suspected appendicitis should undergo laparoscopy? *Br. Med. J.* **296**:1363–4.

11 Pier A, Götz F and Bacher C (1991) Laparoscopic appendectomy in 625 cases: from innovation to routine. *Surg. Laparosc. Endosc.* **1**:8–13.

12 Valla JS, Limonne B, Valla V *et al.* (1991) Laparoscopic appendectomy in children: Report of 465 cases. *Surg. Laparosc. Endosc.* **1**:166–72.

13 Hasson HM (1971) Modified instrument and method for laparoscopy. *Am. J. Obstet. Gynecol.* **110**:886–7.

14 Engström L and Fenyö G (1985) Appendectomy: assessment of stump invagination versus simple ligation. *Br. J. Surg.* **27**:971–2.

15 Sunderland GT, Chisholm EM, San WY, Cheung SCS and Li AKC (1992) Laparoscopic repair of perforated peptic ulcer. *Br. J. Surg.* **79**:785.

16 Leape L and Ramenofsky ML (1980) Laparoscopy for questionable appendicitis. *Ann. Surg.* **191**:410–13.

17 Deutsch A, Zelikovsky A and Reiss R (1982) Laparoscopy in the prevention of unnecessary appendectomies: a prospective study. *Br. J. Surg.* **69**:336–7.

18 Clarke PJ, Hands LJ and Gough MH (1986) The use of laparoscopy in the management of right iliac fossa pain. *Ann. R. Coll. Surg. Engl.* **68**:68–9.

19 Whitworth CM, Whitworth PW and Sanfillipo J (1988) Value of diagnostic laparoscopy in young women with possible appendicitis. *Surg. Gynecol. Obstet.* **167**:187–90.

20 Attwood SE, McGrath J and Hill AD (1992) Laparoscopic approach to Meckel's diverticulectomy. *Br. J. Surg.* **79**:211.

21 Se-Yuan L, Leighton T and Davis I (1991) Prospective analysis of cardiopulmonary responses to laparoscopic cholecystectomy. *J. Laparoendosc. Surg.* **1**:241–6.

22 Wittgen MC (1991) Analysis of the hemodynamic and ventilatory effects of laparoscopic cholecystectomy. *Arch. Surg.* **126**:997–1001.

23 Schreiber JH (1990) Laparoscopic appendectomy in pregnancy. *Surg. Endosc.* **4**:100–2.

24 Redick EJ (1991) Laparoscopic appendectomy. In: Zucker KA (ed.) *Surgical laparoscopy*. Quality Medical Publishing, St Louis.

6

Laparoscopic and Hernioscopic Diagnosis and Repair of Abdominal Wall Hernias

LOTHAR W. POPP

'*Not only must the operation be in no way complicated, but it must be simplified to the utmost.*' Lawson Tait (1845–1899), FRCS, Professor of Gynaecology at Queen's College, Birmingham, UK, made this statement a hundred years ago with respect to the operative treatment of abdominal wall hernias[1]. Today, it is the basic principle of minimal access endoscopic surgery and may be looked upon as the 'categorical imperative'.

Tait definitely preferred diagnosis of hernias from 'within': '*I have an impression that the radical cure of a hernia, other than umbilical, will by and by, be undertaken by abdominal section. A perfect and accurate diagnosis will be made just as soon as the finger in the abdomen reaches the internal aperture of the canal; and this accurate diagnosis is, I may say, a matter of the utmost importance. If the case be one of protrusion, I think there cannot be a doubt that replacement of the viscera can be far more safely affected by traction from within than by pressure from without.*'[1]

Tait's therapeutic approach to abdominal wall hernias from 'within' also deserves careful consideration for modern application: '*Two common glover's sewing needles armed with one piece of salmon silkworm gut are fastened in some convenient needle holder at a very slight angle to one another, so that their points completely coincide, and can be made to enter through one hole in the skin. The left forefinger covers or occupies the inner aperture of the sac, the needles are made to enter from without, and are then separated. The outer needle is then made to dip deeply into the external column of the ring, and the inner needle similarly into the inner column. The needles are then pulled out through the central incision, and as many sutures as may be thought desirable are inserted in this way. When the insertion of the stitches is completed, they can be tied from within and cut short.*'[1] As abdominal section is currently being replaced to a large extent by endoscopy, and laparoscopic instruments are taking the role of the abdominally palpating finger, it is obvious that detailed diagnosis of the hernial sac, removal of its contents and hernia repair are best done by endoscopic surgery.

Abdominal wall hernia repair is the most frequent surgical intervention in the abdomen[2]. Almost half a million procedures are carried out in the USA each year[3]. Table 6.1 shows the number of hernia repairs, cholecystectomies, and appendicectomies in the USA and Germany[4]. The application of modern surgical endoscopy has made appendicectomy[5-7] and cholecystectomy[8-10] routinely used endoscopic procedures. Abdominal wall hernia repair is the next challenge for widespread application of minimal access endoscopic surgery.

Operation	USA (1983)	West Germany (1989)
	Number of operations per 100 000 inhabitants	
Hernia repair	244	209
Cholecystectomy	203	126
Appendicectomy	118	150

Table 6.1: Incidence of the most frequent surgical interventions in the abdomen[4].

In 1989, Bogolavjensky[11] showed the first videotapes on laparoscopic hernia repair in inguinal and femoral hernias. The peritoneum of the hernial sac was opened under endoscopic vision, the musculofascial defect was bluntly dissected, and subsequently filled with rolled-up Vicryl mesh. In early 1990, Popp[12] reported the endoscopic closure of direct inguinal hernia in a female patient by endoscopic suturing of the inner inguinal ring and subsequent intraperitoneal fixation of a dura mater patch using catgut endosutures with extra corporeal knotting technique[13]. Ger et al.[14-16] performed laparoscopic closure of the inner inguinal ring in indirect and direct inguinal hernias using the 'herniastat' for the application of steel clips. Schultz et al.[17] reported on the laser-laparoscopic occlusion of hernias in 20 male patients. The musculofascial defect was closed by preperitoneal implantation of polypropylene mesh. Later in 1990, Popp[18-20] described the improvement of endoscopic hernioplasty by transcutaneous aquadissection of the musculofascial defect and subsequent endoscopic preperitoneal patch repair.

Laparoscopic diagnosis of hernias

As abdominal wall hernias are protrusions from the abdominal cavity, proper diagnosis is best made laparoscopically. We employ laparoscopic technique as described by Semm[13] for all diagnostic and operative endoscopic procedures in the abdominal cavity.

The patient is under general anaesthestic and intubated. Depending upon the extent and localization of the endoscopic procedure, epidural or local anaesthesia are also possible. The abdominal wall is carefully disinfected and draped in the same manner as for laparotomy. We do not shave the pubic hair. We are, however, particularly cautious about preoperative cleansing of the umbilicus. A Foley catheter is inserted into the urinary bladder and the patient is placed in a 15° Trendelenburg position. Pneumoperitoneum with carbon dioxide is established using a Verres needle[21], which is introduced into the base of the umbilicus without incising the skin. In cases of umbilical hernias, the Verres needle is preferably introduced into the left abdominal flank or, in female patients, in the posterior vaginal fornix.

The umbilical trocar is introduced using the Z-technique described by Semm[13]. In patients with previous abdominal surgery, and in all suspicious cases for intra-abdominal adhesions, the 'blind' introduction of the first trocar is carried out under vision of an optic in the perforating trocar sheath: the trocar's tip is first introduced only into the rectus muscle. The trocar is removed and the sheath, which is steadily held with one hand, is connected to the carbon dioxide insufflator set at 12 mmHg maximal intracorporeal pressure. An optic is introduced into the sheath and penetration of the posterior rectus fascia and the peritoneum is carried out under vision by gently turning the trocar sheath and pushing it down towards the pneumoperitoneum[22].

An 11 mm umbilical trocar sheath holding a 30° optic is used for operations at the abdominal wall. In case of umbilical hernia, insertion of the optic trocar in the left abdominal flank can be recommended. The pneumoperitoneum is constantly maintained at 12 mmHg by an electronically controlled carbon dioxide insufflator[13]. The hernial protrusion is endoscopically visualized (see Figure 6.1). When visceral incarceration is present, the contents of the hernial sac can be removed with the use of endoscopic instruments. For laparoscopic repair of an inguinal hernia, a contralateral suprapubic 5 mm trocar insertion and an ipsilateral 5 mm trocar insertion lateral to the umbilicus can be advised (see Figure 6.2).

Laparoscopy allows for extensive inspection of the abdominal wall and also of the contents of the abdominal cavity. By moving the operation table head-down, head-up, or to either side, even hidden abdominal protrusions are accessible to accurate laparoscopic diagnosis. Visualization of the inguinal fossae and the Hesselbach[23] triangles is easy in almost every case. The 10 mm optic or an endoscopic instrument can be introduced into the hernial protrusion in order to estimate the diameter of the internal hernial ring, the depth of the hernial sac, and also the subcutaneous thickness of the abdominal wall. When first doing so, one will be surprised by the very close proximity of the tip of the endoscopic instrument in the hernial sac and the abdominally palpating finger.

Aquadissection of abdominal wall hernias

In hernias with a sliding peritoneum, eg direct inguinal hernias, dissection of the preperitoneal abdominal wall herniation can be carried out by

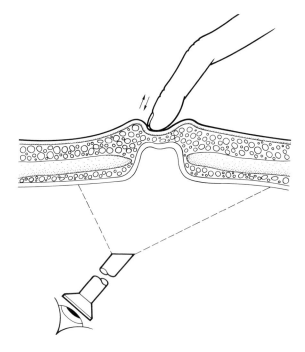

Figure 6.1: Laparoscopic visualization of abdominal wall hernia.

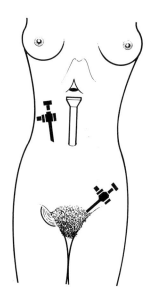

Figure 6.2: Trocar insertions for laparoscopic repair of a right-sided inguinal hernia.

preperitoneal injection of a fluid medium such as physiological saline solution. This modality of blunt dissection of an anatomical space is known as aqua- or hydrodissection.

An injection-set can be used for laparoscopic transperitoneal puncturing and instillation of physiological saline solution (laparoscopic aquadissection). An even easier approach is transcutaneous aquadissection, using an injection cannula which is connected by a plastic tube to a syringe in the hands of

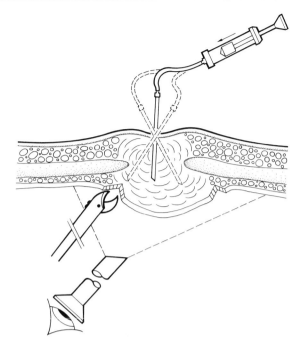

Figure 6.3: Transcutaneous aquadissection of the preperitoneal hernial protrusion. The peritoneum is incised for preperitoneal patch repair (*see also* Figures 6.9 – 6.11).

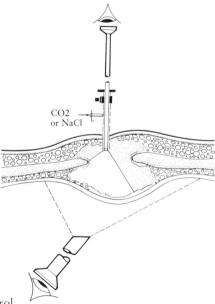

CO2
or NaCl

Figure 6.4: Hernioscopy under laparoscopic control.

the assisting nurse. The injection needle is introduced through the skin on top of the hernial protrusion. The needle tip is identified laparoscopically in the preperitoneal space. As the surgeon manipulates the needle tip, and the nurse simultaneously injects the physiological saline solution, the hernial sac is inverted and the peritoneum is undermined around the internal hernial ring (*see* Figure 6.3). For the inversion of a middle-sized direct inguinal hernial sac, as much as 100–300 ml of physiological saline solution may be needed[18–20].

Hernioscopy

The preperitoneal abdominal wall herniation can be dissected and simultaneously visualized by hernioscopy. A trocar sheath holding an optic is introduced into the subcutaneous fat through a skin incision on top of the hernial protrusion. By creating a subcutaneous (which is at the same time a preperitoneal) emphysema using the carbon dioxide insufflator, or an oedema of physiological saline solution, the peritoneum of the hernial sac is pushed towards the abdominal cavity. The musculofascial defect is gently explored with the tip of the trocar sheath, with which one can palpate the resistance of the intact abdominal wall and the non-resistant gap in the abdominal wall.

We have performed hernioscopy of direct inguinal hernia using a 5 mm hernioscope trocar sheath with a 30° optic for direct vision, and a 10 mm umbilical optic for video-laparoscopic control. In this manner, simultaneous intra- and preperitoneal access to abdominal wall herniation can be achieved (*see* Figures 6.4 and 6.5).

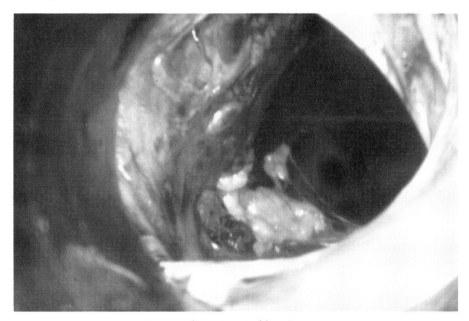

Figure 6.5: Hernioscopic view into direct inguinal hernia.

Hernia repair

Suture repair of the hernial defect which is carried out in a variety of techniques, for instance as described by Bassini[24,25], is known as 'herniorrhaphy'. At 'hernioplasty' or 'hernia patch repair', prosthetic patch material is used for the occlusion of the musculofascial defect[26,27]. At the beginning of the twentieth century, Witzel[28] and Goepel[29] used woven silver wire mesh to close hernial defects. Since then various non-resorbable materials have been applied at hernioplasty: tantalum gauze[30,31], Dacron mesh[27,32], polypropylene mesh (Marlex)[17,33,34], Mersilene mesh[35,36], and polytetrafluoroethylene patch material (expanded PTFE = Gore-Tex)[37–41]. Lichtenstein *et al.*[26] first used the term 'tension-free hernioplasty' with respect to patch repair without the '*suturing together, under tension, of structures that are not normally in apposition*'.

In 1986, Rignault[27] compared his results of 767 hernioplasties and 1382 herniorrhaphies. Particularly effective was the application of hernioplasty in cases of recurrent hernia. In a period of observation lasting more than 14 years, only three of 239 cases (1.2%) recurred again. Rignault recommended a Pfannenstiel incision[42] and preperitoneal implantation of Dacron mesh.

Non-resorbable patch materials have the advantage of covering the musculofascial defect permanently in conjunction with the induction of scar formation around the implant. However, permanent implants may lead to secondary complications such as sequestration and infection. Resorbable patch material, eg Vicryl mesh[18–20] or Vicryl pillow[43–45] was used for 'induction of stabilization of the abdominal wall'[18,19]. Due to induction of extensive scar formation by the gradually resolving patch material, sufficient occlusion of the musculofascial defect can be achieved and the possible disadvantages of a permanent implant can be avoided. More than 6000 Vicryl pillows have been implanted so far during Bassini procedures[44].

Laparoscopic herniorrhaphy

Suturing of the internal hernial ring

In our first cases of repair of indirect and direct inguinal hernia, we used endoscopic suturing techniques for the occlusion of the internal hernial ring[12,19]. For closure of the aperture of an open processus vaginalis peritonei (Nuck's canal), endoscopic suturing with intracorporeal knotting[13] is the most elegant approach. The skilled endoscopic surgeon will put in the necessary stitches carefully, avoiding the spermatic cord in males and including the round ligament in female patients (*see* Figure 6.6). In 1991, Pier *et al.*[46] reported on the closure of the orifice of an indirect inguinal hernia in a male patient using a running endoscopic suture and intracorporeal knotting technique.

Endoscopic suturing with the extracorporeal knotting technique[13] allows strong suture materials to be used in cases of larger abdominal wall herniations. We have applied this method for the apposition of the peritoneum of the

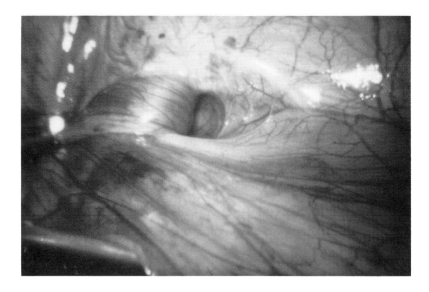

Figure 6.6: Laparoscopic view of a right-sided indirect inguinal hernia in a female patient.

internal ring in direct inguinal hernia[12], for the occlusion of umbilical hernia, and also for repair of fascial defects after extensive adhesiolysis between the abdominal wall and broadly adherent bowel loops. However, the conventional extracorporeal Roeder knot may slip open when the fascial edges are adapted under tension. In these cases, we have used a sixfold fisherman's knot for each suture, and a close distance of about 5 mm between the stitches.

Combination of transcutaneous and endoscopic herniorrhaphy

Hernias in which the peritoneum is fixed to the abdominal wall, eg umbilical and incisional hernias, can be operated by combined transcutaneous and endoscopic herniorrhaphy. The described method is very similar to Tait's procedure cited above[1].

The hernia is visualized endoscopically and the viscera are removed if necessary. A 2 mm skin incision is made lateral to the herniation, and a narrow tunnel to the fascia is formed through the subcutaneous fat using a thin and blunt instrument. A long straight needle with an atraumatic, strong, and non-resorbable suture is inserted through the skin incision and the subcutaneous tunnel so that its tip penetrates the fascia and peritoneum of the hernial sac close to the internal hernial ring. The needle is taken over by an endoscopic needle holder, and three stitches are subsequently made endoscopically: one through the peritoneum in the base of the hernial sac, one deeply through the opposite side of the hernial ring, and one through the abdominal peritoneum next to the hernial ring and back through the abdominal skin incision (*see* Figure 6.7). As many sutures as may be thought desirable are inserted in this way. When the insertion of the stitches is completed, they can be tied to the bases of the subcutaneous tunnels and cut short (*see* Figure 6.8).

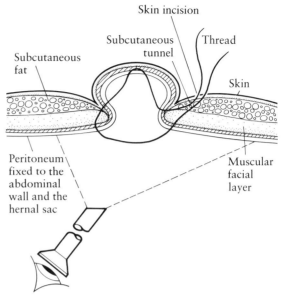

Figure 6.7: Herniorrhaphy in umbilical hernia by combined transcutaneous and endoscopic suture.

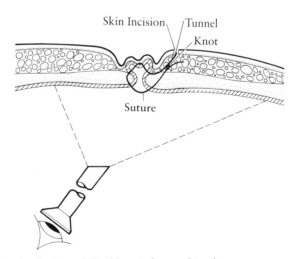

Figure 6.8: Final situs after herniorrhaphy in umbilical hernia by combined transcutaneous and endoscopic suture.

Stapling of the internal hernial ring

Ger *et al.*[14–16] have developed an endoscopic stapling system, the 'herniastat', for the apposition of the internal hernial margins in the first step, and the application of steel clips for hernial occlusion in the second step. The herniastat requires the insertion of a 12 mm trocar sheath, and is capable of delivering eight steel clips. After promising results in long-term animal experience, it is currently being used in clinical trials[16].

Resection of the hernial sac followed by herniorrhaphy

Schultz *et al.*[17] have resected the peritoneum of the hernial sac at the internal ring opening by laser laparoscopy. After dissection of the preperitoneal hernial sac, hernioplasty and subsequent stapling of the resected peritoneal edges were performed. In 30 operated patients, one recurrence has occurred in an eight-month observation period[47].

Laparoscopic hernioplasty

Intraperitoneal hernia patch repair

Laparoscopic intraperitoneal hernia patch repair using a dura mater transplant, which was fixed to the peritoneum by sutures, was reported by Popp[12]. The procedure was carried out in addition to laparoscopic herniorrhaphy in a direct inguinal hernia. During a 19-month follow-up there was no recurrence or other clinical signs.

Intraperitoneal obliteration of the hernial sac

Reich obliterated the hernial sac by inserting a plug of rolled-up polypropylene mesh, with subsequent apposition of the internal hernial ring using endo-sutures[47]. Pier *et al.*[45] used fibrine glue for the obliteration of an open Nuck's canal in a male patient, while Popp[19,20] has tried to achieve obliteration by alterating the peritoneum of the canal using biopsy forceps. The internal inguinal ring was closed in each case by endoscopic sutures. According to Ger's experience[16], it is most likely that obliteration of the open processus vaginalis peritonei will occur without any additional therapeutic means after surgical occlusion of the internal hernial ring.

Preperitoneal hernia patch repair

Laparoscopic preperitoneal hernia patch repair was carried out by Popp[18–20]. After transcutaneous aquadissection of the preperitoneal hernial sac, blunt dissection of this space was performed laparoscopically using four small peritoneal incisions, and resorbable mesh was spread out to cover the musculofascial defect (*see* Figures 6.9 to 6.11). Fixation of the patch material was not considered to be necessary, because the implant is trapped as soon as the pneumoperitoneum is removed. In seven such operated cases, during a two- to 14-month period of observation, there was relief of clinical symptoms and no sign of any recurrence.

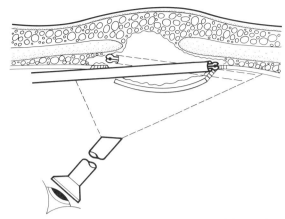

Figure 6.9: Blunt laparoscopic dissection of the aquadissected preperitoneal hernial sac using atraumatic forceps (*see* Figure 6.3).

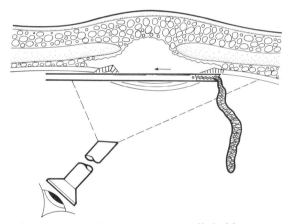

Figure 6.10: A patch is pulled into the preperitoneal space using a needle holder.

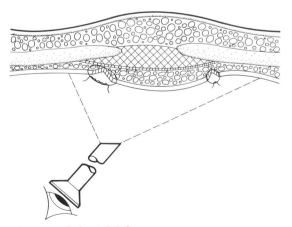

Figure 6.11: A patch is placed on the musculofascial defect.

Preperitoneal stuffing of the hernial sac

Rolled-up patch materials are used for laparoscopic preperitoneal stuffing of the hernial sac[11,17] after it has been opened and dissected laparoscopically. A roll of patch material represents a three-dimensional mesh, which may be even more advantageous for induction of scar formation in the musculofascial defect than a single layer patch. Up to now, only laparoscopic stuffing with rolls of non-resorbable patch materials has been reported.

Hernioscopic hernioplasty

Stuffing of the preperitoneal hernial sac is much easier to perform with the hernioscopic technique than with the laparoscopic approach. It is at the same time an almost atraumatic procedure. After hernioscopic dissection, as described above, the preperitoneal hernial space is stuffed with resorbable patch material through the hernioscopic trocar sheath: an applicator is filled with patch material and passed through the 5 mm hernioscopic trocar sheath. The movements of the tip of the trocar sheath, with the applicator in it, are followed laparoscopically. When the tip is in an appropriate position, the patch material is pushed through the applicator into the preperitoneal space using a 3 mm endoscopic needle holder (*see* Figure 6.12).

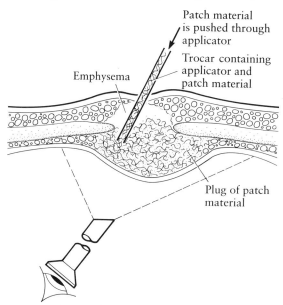

Figure 6.12: Hernioscopic hernioplasty. Patch material is stuffed into the preperitoneal hernial sac.

As the pieces of patch material which can be loaded into the applicator are limited in size, several stuffing procedures are necessary for the creation of a plug of reasonable volume. The growth of the preperitoneal plug is monitored by the laparoscope. For two reasons, care should be taken that the preperitoneal space around the internal hernial ring is sufficiently stuffed.

First, in order to avoid extrusion of the plug by intra-abdominal pressure when it has been stuffed into place, it must be bigger in diameter than the musculofascial defect. Secondly, there must be a circular overlap between the internal hernial ring and the formation of scarring which gradually replaces the plug for 'induced stabilization' of the abdominal wall.

After removal of the preperitoneal carbon dioxide gas emphysema, and also the 5 mm trocar sheath, hernioscopic hernioplasty is completed without having used any suture. With increasing experience and refinement in this minimal access endoscopic procedure, hernioscopic hernioplasty can certainly be performed in appropriate cases without laparoscopic control and under local anaesthesia.

Three female patients with direct inguinal hernias on whom we operated in this way experienced practically no postoperative pain and could have been dismissed from hospital the same day. In one patient we recommended the use of a truss for a two-week period. The other two patients were advised to refrain from sports and from lifting heavy weights for six weeks. In a two- to four-month follow-up period, no recurrences of inguinal pain or herniation have occurred.

Discussion

Clinical experience in minimal access endoscopic surgery of abdominal wall hernias is still limited. In the University Clinic for Women in Kiel, Germany, 14 endoscopic hernia repairs have been carried out since 1989, including indirect and direct inguinal hernia, umbilical and incisional hernia. As our department under Professor Kurt Semm can look back on the development of pelviscopic surgery over more than 20 years, during which almost 19 000 pelviscopic procedures have been carried out, we feel that our experience can also be applied to the new field of endoscopic hernia repair. Hernia repair has been performed only in female patients scheduled for gynaecological pelviscopic surgery. The age of the patients ranged from 27 to 69 years. So far we have seen no recurrent hernia.

We believe that some female patients presenting with chronic pelvic pain suffer from abdominal wall herniations rather than from gynaecological disease. Therefore, when taking the patient's history, we are now much more specific about questions concerning the type of pain. Sharp inguinal pain on one side, when playing tennis for instance, leads one to suspect the presence of inguinal hernia. At laparoscopy the inguinal fossae are carefully inspected while the abdominal wall is palpated in the inguinal areas. Some cases, out of the roughly 20% of laparoscopically unexplained pelvic pain in women, may thus be diagnosed as abdominal wall hernias. Endoscopic repair of the hernia is performed during the same operation.

Different methods of endoscopic hernia repair have been used since 1989. According to Tait[1], the least complicated operations always prove to be best. In hernias with a sliding peritoneum, eg direct inguinal hernias, transcutaneous aquadissection is the least invasive way for the dissection of the preperitoneal hernial sac. The least traumatic hernia repair in this case is hernioscopic hernioplasty. Further clinical studies must evaluate how large a musculofascial defect can be for induction of stabilization of the abdominal wall by means of preperitoneal implantation of resorbable patch material to reveal satisfactory long-term results.

Apposition of the internal hernial ring with steel staples may currently be the easiest method for laparoscopic occlusion of indirect inguinal hernia. The disadvantages of permanent steel staples may be overcome by the development of appropriate resorbable clips. Endoscopic suturing techniques are, however, an excellent alternative in the hands of the skilled endoscopic surgeon. A combined transcutaneous and endoscopic suturing technique for the occlusion of umbilical and incisional hernias, in which the peritoneum is fixed to the hernial sac wall, is another promising approach which may be improved by including resorbable patch material into the sutures.

The long periods of convalescence after conventional hernia repair are caused by incision and re-apposition of skin, subcutaneous fat and fascia. Operating on skin and fat does not add at all to the postoperative stability of the abdominal wall. Suturing the musculofascial layers together under tension certainly causes postoperative pain, but does not necessarily lead to better success of the intervention compared to 'tension-free hernioplasty'.

Minimal access endoscopic surgery will clearly play a beneficial part in the repair of abdominal wall hernias. Skin incisions are minimized and preperitoneal dissection of the hernial sac is done atraumatically by aquadissection or hernioscopy. Repair of the musculofascial defect is preferably done by hernioplasty, and by stapling or suturing the internal hernial ring only. In appropriate cases, endoscopic hernia repair may become an out-patient procedure which can be carried out under local anaesthesia.

As a consequence, minimal access endoscopic hernia repair will reduce postoperative pain and also shorten the period of convalescence dramatically. When applying these possible benefits to the most frequently performed surgical intervention in the abdomen, one can expect a reduction in the cost of medical care and a substantial improvement in the postoperative well-being of patients.

References

1 Tait L (1891) A discussion on treatment of hernia by median abdominal section. *Br. Med. J.* 2:685–7.

2 Nyhus LM and Bombeck CT (1977) Hernias. In: Sabiston DC (ed.) *Textbook of surgery, the biological basis of modern surgical practice.* WB Saunders Company, Philadelphia.

3 US Department of Health, Education and Welfare (1974) *National Health Survey – surgical operations in short-stay hospitals, United States – 1971.* Series 13, No. 18, Nov. 1974.

4 Siewert JR, Bollschweiler E and Hempel K (1990) Wandel der Eingriffshäufigkeit in der Allgemeinchirurgie. *Chirurg.* 61:855–63.

5   Semm K (1982) Advances in pelviscopic surgery. Current problems in obstetrics and gynecology. *Obstet. Gynecol.* **10**:7–42.

6   Semm K (1983) Die endoskopische Appendektomie. *Gynaekol. prax.* **7**:131–40.

7   Semm K (1991) Technische Operationsschritte der endoskopischen Appendektomie. *Langenbecks. Arch. Chir.* **376**:121–6.

8   Mühe E (1986) Die erste Cholecystektomie durch das Laparoskop. *Langenb. Arch. Chir.* **369**:804.

9   Mühe E (1990) Laparoskopische Cholecystektomie. *Endoskopie heute* **4**:262–6.

10 Perissat J, Collet D and Belliard R (1990) Gallstones: laparoscopic treatment – cholecystectomy, cholecystostomy, and lithotripsy. *Surg. Endosc.* **4**:1–5.

11 Bogolavjensky S (1989) *Laparoscopic treatment of inguinal and femoral hernia* (video presentation). 18th Annual Meeting of the American Association of Gynecologic Laparoscopists. Washington DC.

12 Popp LW (1990) Endoscopic patch repair of inguinal hernia in a female patient. *Surg. Endosc.* **4**:10–12.

13 Semm K (1984) *Operationslehre für endoskopische Abdominal-Chirurgie / Operative Pelviskopie / Operative Laparoskopie.* Schattauer, Stuttgart.

14 Ger R (1982) The management of certain abdominal herniae by intra-abdominal closure of the neck of the sac. *Ann. R. Coll. Surg. Eng.* **64**:342–4.

15 Ger R, Monroe K, Duvivier R and Mischrick A (1990) Management of indirect inguinal hernia by a laparoscopic closure of the neck of the sac. *Am. J. Surg.* **159**:370–3.

16 Ger R (1991) Laparoskopische Hernienoperationen. *Chirurg.* **62**:266–70.

17 Schultz L, Graber J, Pietrafitta J and Hickok D (1990) Laser laparoscopic herniorrhaphy: a clinical trial – preliminary results. *J. Laparoendosc. Surg.* **1**:41–5.

18 Popp LW (1990) Endoskopischer Verschluss einer Leistenhernie / Hernioplastic inguinale par coelioscopie. In: Semm K, Bernard P and Mettler L, eds. *Geburtshilfe und Gynäkologie in Deutschland und Frankreich / Gynécologie et obstétrique en France et en Allemagne.* 70–81.

19 Popp LW (1991) Improvement in endoscopic hernioplasty: transcutaneous aquadissection of the musculo-fascial defect, and pre-peritoneal endoscopic patch repair. *J. Laparoendosc. Surg.* **1**:83–90.

20 Popp LW (1991) Endoskopische Hernioplastik. *Chirurg.* **62**:336–9.

21 Veress J (1938) Ein neues Instrument zur Ausführung von Brust- und Bauchpunktionen und Pneumothoraxbehandlung. *Dtsch. med. Woschr.* **41**:1480.

22 Semm K (1988) Sichtkontrollierte Peritoneumperforation zur operativen Pelviskopie. *Geburtsh. Frauenheilk.* **48**:436–9.

23 Hesselbach FK (1814) *Neueste anatomische-pathologische Untersuchungen über den Ursprung und das Fortschreiten der Leisten- und Schenkelbrüche.* Stahel, Würzburg. 1–72.

24 Bassini E (1887) Nuovo metodo per la cura radicale dell'ernia. *Atti. Cong. Ass. Med. Ital.* **2**:179.

25 Bassini E (1889) Nuovo metodo operativo per la cura dell'ernia inguinale. *R. Stabilimento Prosperini Padova* 1–103.

26 Lichtenstein IJ, Shulman AG, Amid PK and Motillor MM (1989) The tension-free hernioplasty. *Am. J. Surg.* **157**:188–93.

27 Rignault DP (1986) Properitoneal prosthetic inguinal hernioplasty through a Pfannenstiel approach. *Surg. Gynecol. Obstet.* **163**:465–8.

28 Witzel O (1900) Über den Verschluß von Bauchwunden und Bruchpforten durch versenkte Silberdrahtnetze (Einheilung von Filgranpelotten). *Centralbl. Chir.* **27**:257–60.

29 Goepel R (1900) Über die Verschließung von Bruchpforten durch Einheilung geflochtener, fertiger Silberdrahtnetze (Silberdrahtpelotten). *Verh. Dsch. Ges. Chir.* **29**:174-7.

30 Koontz AR (1948) Preliminary report on the use of tantalum mesh in the repair of ventral hernias. *Ann. Surg.* **127**:1079–85.

31 Lam CR, Szilagyi DE and Puppendahl M (1948) Tantalum gauze in the repair of large postoperative ventral hernias. *Arch. Surg.* **57**:234–44.

32 Wolstenholme JT (1956) Use of commercial Dacron fabric in the repair of inguinal hernias and abdominal wall defects. *A.M.A. Arch. Surg.* **73**:1004–8.

33 Usher FC (1963) Hernia repair with knitted polypropylene mesh. *Surg. Gynecol. Obstet.* **117**:239–40.

34 Usher FC (1978) Hernia repair with Marlex mesh. In: Nyhus LM and Condon RE, eds. *Hernias.* JB Lippincott Company, Philadelphia.

35 Calne RY (1978) Buttressing of the inguinal wall with prosthetic material: repair of bilateral groin hernias with Mersilene mesh behind the rectus abdominis muscle. In: Nyhus LM and Condon RE, eds. *Hernias.* JB Lippincott Company, Philadelphia.

36 Notaras MJ (1978) Experience with Mersilene mesh in abdominal wall repair. In: Nyhus LM and Condon RE, eds. *Hernias.* JB Lippincott Company, Philadelphia.

37 Bauer JJ, Salky BA, Gelernt IM and Kreel I (1987) Repair of large abdominal wall defects with expanded polytetrafluoroethylene (PTFE). *Ann. Surg.* **206**:765–9.

38 Hamer-Hodges DW and Scott NB (1985) Replacement of an abdominal wall defect using expanded PTFE sheet (Gore-Tex). *J. R. Coll. Surg. Edinb.* **30**:65-7.

39 Lei B van der, Bleichbrodt RP, Simmermacher RKJ and Schilfgaarde R van (1989) Expanded polytetrafluoroethylene patch for the repair of large abdominal wall defects. *Br. J. Surg.* **76**:803–5.

40 Pailler JL, Manaa J, Vicq PH, Brissiaud JC and Gandon F (1987) Cure des hernies de l'aine avec interposition d'une prothèse de PTFE (à propos des 185 premières plaques mises en place dans le service). *Lettre Chirurgicale (Lille)* **55**:13–15.

41 Wool NL, Straus AK and Roseman DL (1985) Clinical experience with the Gore-Tex Soft Tissue Patch in hernia repair: a preliminary report. *Proc. Inst. Med. Chgo.* **38**:33.

42 Pfannenstiel J (1899) Über die Vortheile des suprasymphysären Fascienquerschnittes für die gynäkologischen Köeliotomien, zugleich ein Beitrag zu der Indikationsstellung der Operationswege. In: Volkmann R, ed. *Sammlung klinischer Vorträge*. Breitkopf und Härtel, Leipzig.

43 Brenner J (1990) Vicryl Kissen – induzierte Stabilität im Leistenbereich. *Ethicon-op-forum* **142**:1–15.

44 Lierse W and Brenner J (1991) Die Implantation des Vicryl Kissens bei der Herniotomie – induzierte Stabilität im Leistenbereich. Serie: *Im Dienste der Chirurgie, Ethicon* **78**:2–11.

45 Willmen HR (1987) Die 'Wende' in der Therapie von Inguinal- und Hiatushernien durch Induktion tragfähigen Narbengewebes. *Chirurg.* **58**:300–2.

46 Pier A, Götz F and Thevissen P (1991) Laparoskopische Versorgung einer indirekten Inguinalhernie (Fallbeschreibung). *Endoskopie heute* **1**:13–16.

47 Salerno GM, Fitzgibbons RJ and Filipi CJ (1991) Laparoscopic inguinal hernia repair. In: Zucker KA, ed. *Surgical laparoscopy*. Quality Medical Publishing, St Louis.

7

Laparoscopic Hernia Repair

MAURICE E. ARREGUI and JORGE L. NAVARRETE

Introduction

With the remarkable success of laparoscopic cholecystectomy, it is worth looking at another common general surgical problem such as inguinal hernias (500 000 of which are repaired annually in the United States)[1] to see if the techniques of minimal access surgery can confer the same advantages of reduced pain, quicker recovery, and improved cosmesis while maintaining a low complication rate. Moreover, using tensionless technique with mesh reinforcement, it seems reasonable to postulate that the repairs will be superior and less likely to recur than classic open anterior hernia repairs, which have a recurrence rate of 0–7 % for indirect, 1–10 % for direct, and 5–35 % for recurrent hernias[2]. Unlike with laparoscopic cholecystectomy, the cost of laparoscopic herniorrhaphy is probably higher than that of the standard anterior approach. This is due to increased equipment costs, the need for general anaesthesia, and (with our own particular technique) added operating-room time. However, there is a potentially shorter recovery time which ought to reduce the economic impact due to loss of productivity.

Technique

The procedure is usually performed on an out-patient basis with general anaesthesia (although we have successfully done one case using an epidural block). Antibiotics are given intravenously on induction of general anaesthesia. After inspecting the peritoneal cavity, the hernia is assessed. If a unilateral or bilateral indirect inguinal hernia or a unilateral direct inguinal hernia is encountered, the preperitoneal space is usually entered by incising the orifice of the hernia sac. If bilateral direct inguinal hernias are encountered,

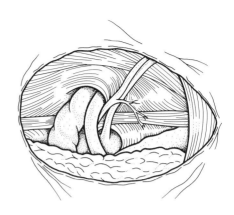

Figure 7.1: Transperitoneal preperitoneal dissection exposes the iliopubic tract, Cooper's ligament, vas deferens, spermatic vessels, transversus abdominis, transversalis fascia, rectus muscle and epigastric vessels. The internal ring, Hesselbach's triangle and the femoral canal (the sites of hernia formation) are exposed. (From Arregui ME *et al.* (1992) Laparoscopic mesh repair of inguinal hernia using a preperitoneal approach: a preliminary approach. *Surg. Laparosc. Endosc.* **2:**1, with permission.)

the whole procedure is usually performed extraperitoneally without incising the peritoneum. Recently, we have started performing all our laparoscopic hernia repairs totally extraperitoneally. Once the preperitoneal space is entered, dissection is carried out to expose the internal ring and surrounding structures, Hesselbach's triangle, the femoral canal and Cooper's ligament (*see* Figure 7.1). A large piece of mesh (10 × 15 cm) covering all the above areas is then secured (on the ileopubic tract with staples or suture, transversus abdominus aponeurosis and transversus abdominis lateral to the internal ring) to prevent slippage and herniation of the mesh into the fascial defect (*see* Figure 7.2). Once the mesh is in place, the peritoneal defects are meticulously closed with suture to prevent herniation of the intraperitoneal contents into the preperitoneal space and to reduce the chances of adhesions associated with disruption of the peritoneum or exposure to prosthetic material[3,4,5].

Rationale for preperitoneal approach

The contemporary literature emphasizes a tensionless approach[6] using mesh, and certainly many would advocate the use of mesh for multiply recurrent or difficult hernia repairs[7,8,9,10,11,12,13]. Lichtenstein and others have demonstrated low infection rates using mesh in many large series, despite the traditional reluctance to use prosthetic material for first-time hernia repairs[7,14]. The preperitoneal approach to inquinal hernias has long been advocated by Nyhus, since the origin of the defect can be directly addressed[13,15]. A laparoscopic approach has the advantage of allowing access to the preperitoneal space without the disadvantage of an open incision, as with the Stoppa or Nyhus approach. Another advantage is that one can work directly at the level of the defect, both to identify the type and extent of the defect clearly, and to reinforce the weak tissues at the proper plane of origin of the defect. Indeed, by placing a large piece of mesh in the preperitoneal space, increased intra-abdominal pressure should apply an evenly distributed force on the peritoneum which pushes the mesh more firmly onto the anterior

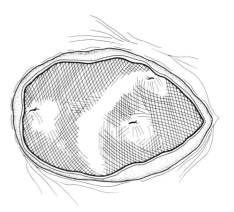

Figure 7.2: Mesh is in place covering all hernia or potential hernia sites. Sutures are on the iliopubic tract, transversus abdominis aponeurosis and transversus abdominis lateral to the internal ring. (From Arregui ME *et al.* (1992) Laparoscopic mesh repair of inguinal hernia using a preperitoneal approach: a preliminary report. *Surg. Laparosc. Endosc.* 2:1, with permission.)

abdominal wall. Suturing or stapling the mesh should prevent slippage or herniation of the mesh through the fascial defect and a possible recurrence due to loss of reinforcement. Although, Stoppa feels that fixation is unnecessary (we have recently stopped fixation of the mesh). The mesh is also large enough to cover all potential sites of herniation in the inquinofemoral region, and could thus prevent future hernias in this area.

Other techniques

Other techniques include clip or suture closure of a small indirect hernia, use of intraperitoneal mesh, and the plug and small patch technique.

Ger has studied ring closure with clips of small and medium-sized indirect inguinal hernias during open surgery and demonstrated no recurrence of these hernias[16]. He has subsequently studied the use of staples for ring closure in beagles again with good results[17]. Recently he performed stapled closure of indirect hernias in man[18]. He has since repaired 31 hernias in 24 patients: 26 indirect hernias, three direct, one femoral, and one recurrent. He has had no intraoperative complications and only one postoperative complication (a case of meralgia paraesthetica). There have been six recurrences. Five were attributed to insufficient, misplaced or ineffective staples, and one was in a sliding incarcerated hernia. The average follow-up is 19 months[19]. The advantages of this technique include the ease and the speed in which it can be performed, the ability to perform it under local anaesthesia, and the avoidance of mesh. The disadvantages include unsuitability for large indirect hernias (and probably direct hernias too), closure under tension which requires restriction of activity, and the approximating of peritoneal tissues which theoretically will not provide a strong scar and predisposes to recurrence.

Rosin, at St Mary's Hospital in London, England, is performing simple inversion of the indirect sac with high ligation. For larger indirect defects, he is suturing the ring closed. He has repaired 57 hernias in 51 patients; 54 were indirect, two were femoral, and there was one spigellian hernia. There have been no intraoperative complications and one postoperative transient hydrocoele. The average follow-up has been 12 months. Patients, including manual labourers, are allowed to return to work a week later without restriction[20].

Spaw uses ring-plasty (or lateral suture closure) for small and medium indirect inguinal hernias. He reports an average operating time of 49.9 minutes in 19 patients. Patients return to work an average of 5.5 days after surgery, and take an average of 4.3 pain pills (7.5 mg hydrocodone bitartrate with 500 mg acetaminophen). He reports no recurrences with the ring closure technique. For all other hernias he uses an intraperitoneal onlay patch of Gortex mesh (WL Gore and Associates Inc, Flagstaff, Arizona) which is stapled onto Cooper's ligament inferior-medially and at the periphery of the patch. With this technique on 19 patients so repaired the average operating time is 61.7 minutes, the time off work averages 5.7 days, and the average number of pain pills taken is 4.5 hydrocodone tablets. He has performed 45 inguinal hernia repairs (22 direct, 21 indirect and one femoral) and one incisional hernia using these two techniques. Operative complications include one laceration of a right inferior epigastric vein and one acute scrotal oedema. There have been three conversions to open surgery. Postoperative complications include one recurrence medial to an onlay patch repair[21,22].

Dion has performed 15 ring closures with zero Prolene suture for type II (Nyhus classification) indirect inguinal hernias. To date, he has had no intraoperative or postoperative complications and no recurrences[23,24]. For all other hernias he uses a preperitoneal approach. Shlain also uses ringplasty or suture closure of the internal ring. Occasionally he will place a small plug of mesh into the orifice of the hernia. He does not take out the sac. To date 58 ring closures have been performed, with no recurrences. Patients are not allowed to lift heavy weights for four weeks afterwards[25].

Franklin attached a large 12 × 15 cm piece of Prolene mesh intraperitoneally with a combination of transfascial suturing and stapling. With this technique, 65 hernias (32 direct and 33 indirect) have been repaired. He reports one recurrence in 63 patients in a follow-up averaging 11 months (range two weeks to 28 months). Intraoperative complications include laceration of the inferior epigastric artery (one case) and inadequate prosthesis size (two cases). Postoperative complications include leg numbness (two cases), haematoma (one case), testicular pain (two cases) and pseudohernias which later resolved (three cases)[26,27]. This approach is easily and rapidly performed, but there is the obvious disadvantage that the prosthetic material in the peritoneal cavity may lead to adhesion formation, with the subsequent risk of small bowel obstruction. Long-term results will be particularly important in these patients.

Fitzgibbons originally stapled Prolene mesh onto the peritoneum for all hernia defects[28]. Because of early failures with direct hernias he now uses intraperitoneal mesh for indirect defects and a preperitoneal mesh repair for the direct defects. With this intraperitoneal onlay mesh technique he has repaired 42 indirect hernias and two direct ones. Both direct hernias have recurred. He describes these as 'retained hernias', since they were apparent immediately following surgery. He attributes this to the complete slippage of the mesh and the loose peritoneum into the direct hernia defect, since the staples were placed only on the peritoneum and not on the fascial tissue. He has also performed 59 transabdominal preperitoneal repairs, with one recurrence[29]. Filipi likewise abandoned the intraperitoneal mesh after two procedures in which he had one recurrence with a repair of a direct hernia. The other hernia was an indirect one. He is currently employing a preperitoneal approach[30].

Schultz reported using a plug of mesh in the hernia orifice, but has modified his technique and now uses a large piece of mesh preperitoneally[31]. Corbitt, who began with a plug and a small piece of mesh, has also modified his approach to a preperitoneal approach with a large piece of mesh[32]. Both reported recurrences resulting from direct defects that had been overlooked.

Indirect hernias are usually readily apparent since they are likely to be congenital due to failed obliteration of the processus vaginalis (although I have had one case with a clinical indirect hernia which was not apparent at laparoscopy unless pressure was applied to the anterior abdominal wall). This probably represented herniated preperitoneal fat or lipoma of the cord. This patient, who had a contralateral indirect hernia which was repaired, is being followed up. If he has significant clinical symptoms, a repair will be performed. Other patients have been operated on for indirect hernias and, during preperitoneal dissection, have been found to have concomitant small direct hernias which were not apparent on intraperitoneal inspection.

One disadvantage of a limited dissection, therefore, is that hernias may be overlooked; another disadvantage is that the small mesh could migrate into the fascial defect. Even in those patients in whom the plug is effective, an unnatural mass effect will be felt. Using his early plug technique, Schultz had eight recurrences in his first 50 patients. He has therefore modified his approach to a more extended transperitoneal dissection of the preperitoneal space, so that concomitant hernias cannot be overlooked. Pieces of mesh are placed in the defect and then the area is covered with a larger mesh measuring 8.5×6.5 cm. Schultz has now performed an additional 150 hernia repairs using this preperitoneal approach, with no recurrences. Of this total of 200 cases, there have been 77 direct, 121 indirect and two femoral hernias. There have been two cases of bleeding. Both were admitted for 24 hours and discharged uneventfully. Two patients developed postoperative small bowel obstruction, and 16 minor complications have occurred, including five urinary retentions, two haematomas, two testicular swellings and three cases of nausea[33]. His first 150 cases resumed normal activity after an average of 2.4 days, and returned to work without restriction after 4.7 days[34]. Corbitt likewise had a 15 % recurrence or missed hernia rate with his original plug and small patch technique[35]. Both have switched to using larger pieces of mesh after a more extensive preperitoneal dissection.

Katkhouda, in Nice, France, also originally started with the plug and mesh technique but, after two recurrences in his first 12 cases, abandoned it for the preperitoneal approach with mesh[36]. Schafmayer's team in Germany have likewise used a plug and patch to repair 92 hernias. There have been two haematomas, two cases of periostial pain and one migration of one of the plugs to the external ring. They report no recurrences or overlooked hernias to date, which they attribute to the fact that most of their repairs have been done on young patients with indirect hernias who would rarely have an associated direct defect. In older patients a vigorous search is always made to look for an associated direct or indirect hernia[37].

MacFadyen, in Houston, Texas, recently reported results of 635 hernia repairs on 563 patients based on a questionnaire of surgeons throughout the United States. This was based on various techniques using intraperitoneal mesh (186), transperitoneal preperitoneal (359) and totally extraperitoneal approaches (90). Overall the average follow-up was 5.6 months. Complications included nine recurrences (1.4 %), 17 haematomas (2.6 %), nine cases of thigh pain (1.4 %), eight cases of emphysema of the scrotum (1.2 %), eight of urinary retention (1.2 %), three of scrotal hydroceles (0.4 %), two bladder injuries (0.3 %), one case of pelvic ostitis (0.15 %), one of abdominal bloating (0.15 %) and one of testicular pain (0.15 %). Of the nine recurrences, six (3.2 %) occurred with the intraperitoneal onlay prosthesis, three (0.84 %) occurred with the transperitoneal preperitoneal approach, and there were none when the totally extraperitoneal approach was used. He also collected data on 89 ring closures and reported a 2.2 % recurrence, while 87 plug and patch repairs had a 6.8 % recurrence. From his review of the collected data, he concluded that: the overall complication rates are low, the plug and patch of the internal ring has a high recurrence rate, and recurrences are more frequent in the early experience of the surgeon. The recurrences are usually due to a small prosthesis and inadequate fixation of the mesh. He also concludes that the best repair technique to date is the placement of a large prosthesis (8–10 × 12–15 cm) either in the peritoneal or preperitoneal space. Moreover, he found that intra-abdominal adhesions have not yet been a major problem[38].

The above techniques need to be studied and understood. There does seem to be a general trend to using a preperitoneal approach with a large piece of mesh. Once laparoscopic herniorrhaphy is well understood and the techniques worked out, individualization of patient circumstances and type of hernia may call for individualization of technique used.

Anatomy of the preperitoneal hernia

Unless surgeons have routinely performed preperitoneal hernia repairs by the open approach, there is a general lack of familiarity with this area. If the approach is totally extraperitoneal through the umbilicus and the proper preperitoneal space is entered, then the anatomy is much as discussed by Stoppa or Nyhus[12,13]. There is a problem, however, if the surgeon does not enter the proper preperitoneal plane. With the magnification, the smaller space, the inability to feel and the different perspective of the laparoscopic technique, the wrong space can be entered and total confusion will result.

The technique can be even more confusing if the entrance to the preperitoneal space is achieved transperitoneally through an incision in the peritoneum at the orifice of an indirect or direct hernia. The problem is that most surgeons do not properly understand the relationships of the transversalis fascial to the fascias associated with the peritoneum.

In the inguinal area, the peritoneum is the deepest layer which is closely adherent to a thin and usually well defined preperitoneal fascia (see Figure 7.3). This poorly described fascia forms a separate layer which can be confused with the transversalis fascia. It is a thin fibrous sheet, which can

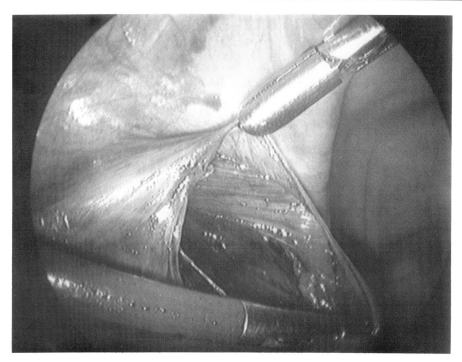

Figure 7.3: The well developed transverse fibres of the preperitoneal fascia can be seen clearly between the peritoneum and the umbilical ligament during the transperitoneal dissection of this indirect left inguinal hernia.

best be seen when magnified laparoscopically, enveloping the peritoneum and following the peritoneal hernial sac into the inguinal canal in both direct and indirect hernias. This preperitoneal sheet also envelops both the vas deferens and the spermatic vessels as they enter the internal ring. Indeed, this forms the inner covering of the cord structures (*see* Figure 7.4). At the orifice of the indirect hernia the fibrous ring surrounding this orifice is often quite strong (*see* Figure 7.5) and may play an important role in ring closure, as in Ger's technique. If the preperitoneal space is entered by incising the peritoneum at the orifice of the indirect hernia, the space between the peritoneum and the preperitoneal fascia is often entered (*see* Figure 7.6). In order to get into the proper plane, the preperitoneal space of dissection, this fascial tissue must be incised medially as well as laterally. When in the proper plane, the preperitoneal fat and loose tissue easily separates from the weak fascial plane surrounding the epigastric vessels and its branches. The proper plane of dissection is just deep to the epigastric vessels in the inguinal area. When the peritoneum, preperitoneal fascia and fat are separated from the pelvic, and anterior abdominal wall, the essential preperitoneal structures forming the inguinal–femoral area can be properly identified (*see* Figure 7.7). The landmarks include Cooper's ligament proceeding laterally from the midline and to beyond the femoral vein where it disappears from the operating field. Above this is the iliopubic tract, which attaches medially to Cooper's ligament and then travels laterally, forming the curvilinear medial boundary of the femoral canal and proceeding around and anterior to the

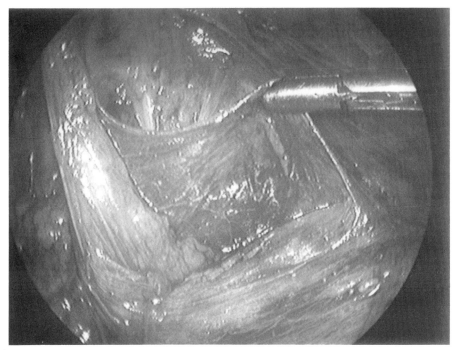

Figure 7.4: The preperitoneal fascia which was completely enveloping the spermatic vessels and vas deferens has been split anteriorly. Note how this is intimately attached to the peritoneum. This was a totally extraperitoneal dissection of a right direct inguinal hernia.

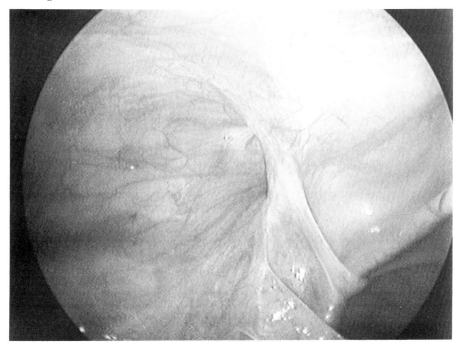

Figure 7.5: The thickened dense tissue forming the medial aspect of the internal inguinal ring of this indirect left inguinal hernia.

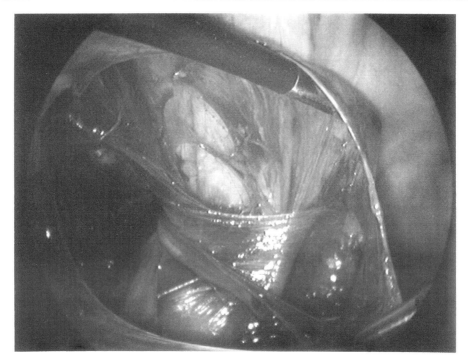

Figure 7.6: In this transperitoneal dissection of a left indirect inguinal hernia, the preperitoneal fascia is between the peritoneum and the medial preperitoneal space. The vas deferens is seen coursing over the umbilical ligament medially and then diving into the orifice of the internal ring.

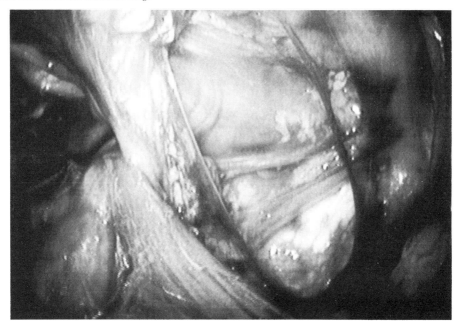

Figure 7.7: In this left inguinal hernia, the internal ring is seen to the left. The epigastric vessels, spermatic vessel bundle and vas are seen laterally. Hesselbach's triangle or inguinal floor, iliopubic tract, and Cooper's ligament are seen medially. (From Arregui ME (1992) Training requirements for laparoscopic hernia repair. *Laparosc. Foc.* 1:1, with permission.)

femoral vein and inferior epigastric vessels, before travelling under the vas deferens and spermatic vessels as they enter the inguinal canal, and finally proceeding laterally to form the inferior border of the internal ring. At this point the origin of the transversus abdominis muscle can be seen as an arch over the inguinal floor and forming the lateral border of the internal ring. As the transversus abdominis muscle proceeds medially, a strong aponeurotic fascia may proceed from the transversus abdominis to form the medial border of the internal ring, extending medially as a strong sheet incorporating the iliopubic tract and inserting onto Cooper's ligament as the inferior portion of the iliopubic tract[39] (see Figures 7.8 and 7.9). Deep to this is a thin tissue of variable strength which is the transversalis fascia. When the projection of the transversus abdominis muscle onto Cooper's ligament is incomplete, the floor is covered by an often thin and transparent transversalis fascia, predisposing to a direct inguinal hernia (see Figure 7.10). The transversalis fascia is part of the endoabdominal fascia covering the abdominal and pelvic cavity. It contributes to the floor of the inguinal canal and forms a sling around the internal ring. The other structures exposed during the dissection of the inguinal preperitoneal space include the transversus abdominis aponeurotic arch, which forms the superior border of Hesselbach's triangle. Medial and deep to this is rectus abdominis muscle. This is also covered on its deep surface by a transversalis fascia which is often so thin that it is barely perceptible during preperitoneal dissection with either open or laparoscopic approaches. The spermatic vessels course in the retroperitoneal space just deep to the peritoneum. The vas deferens emerges from the pelvis medial to the medial umbilical ligament and courses over the external iliac vessels before entering the internal ring, which is made up of transversalis fascia and reinforced by a conglomeration of fascial fibres, composed mainly of the preperitoneal fascia which here is often unusually thick, especially medially (see Figures 7.5 and 7.6). In most cases a thickened band can be seen transperitoneally in both patients with and without an indirect inguinal hernia. This often highly visible band courses laterally, forming the anterior and medial border of the internal ring. Medially and inferiorly it proceeds between the obliterated umbilical artery and the peritoneum. This band is called the transverse vesical fold (see Figure 7.11).

Spaw has coined the term 'triangle of doom' to warn surgeons not to place clips or sutures between the vas deferens and the spermatic artery, because this is the location of the femoral nerve and external iliac artery and vein: I have extended this 'triangle of doom' laterally to the iliopubic tract. This extension then includes the genitofemoral nerve and the lateral femoral cutaneous nerve, which is located just anterior to the iliopsoas muscle and is often not seen during the preperitoneal dissection (see Figure 7.12). A suture or clip placed here could cause nerve injury resulting in painful nerve entrapment syndrome, as can occur with the ilioinguinal and iliohypogastric nerves during anterior approaches.

It is essential to identify the anatomy of the preperitoneal space carefully, to identify the particular pathological anatomy responsible for the particular hernia, and more importantly to perform the preperitoneal repair safely and place the sutures or staples correctly to prevent recurrences (see Figure 7.13).

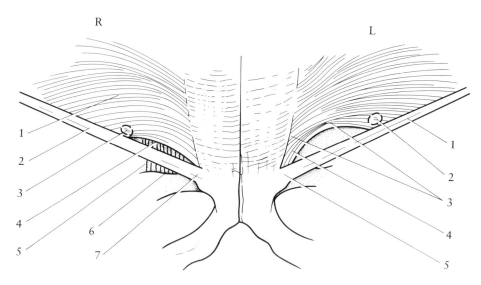

Figure 7.8: Strong inguinal floor on the right; on the left, the inguinal floor is essentially open[15]. (From Lampe EW (1989) Special comment: the anatomy of the inguinal region and its relation to groin hernias. In: Nyhus LM and Condon RE, eds. *Hernia*, 3rd ed. JB Lippincott, Philadelphia, with permission.)

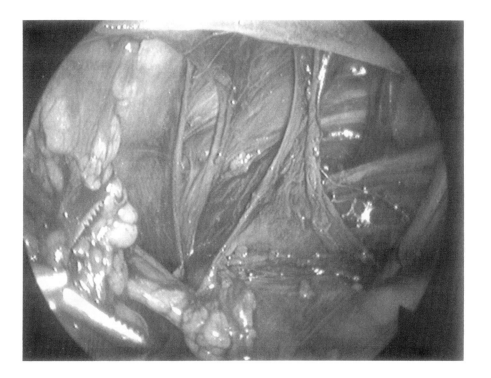

Figure 7.9: On this right inguinal hernia, the medial aspect of the internal orifice shows a very dense strong fascia which is a continuation of the transversus abdominis. On either side the thin fibres of the enveloping transversalis fascia, which has been dissected off, can be seen to be quite thin.

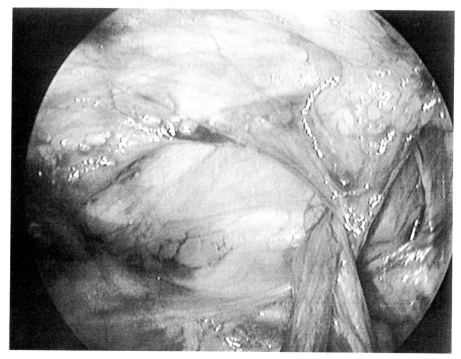

Figure 7.10: Preperitoneal dissection of this left direct inguinal hernia reveals a very thin transparent transversalis fascia forming the medial aspect of the internal ring. The border of the transversus abdominis aponeurotic arch can be clearly seen coursing medially. The direct hernia defect is seen medial to the epigastric vessels and lateral to the rectus abdominis muscle.

Technical details of the preperitoneal repair

After induction of general anaesthesia, the patient is given 1 g of a first or second generation cephalosporin (I usually give 1 g Kefzol, Cefazolin Sodium, Eli Lilly Inc., Indianapolis, Indiana). In addition, 500 mg of cephalothin is mixed in with 500 cc of normal saline for soaking the mesh and for irrigation. A Foley catheter is inserted. With the patient placed in a slightly Trendelenberg position, an incision is made longitudinally in a crease along the inferior portion of the umbilicus. A Verres needle is used for peritoneal insufflation. Once adequate insufflation has been achieved to a pressure of 15 mmHg, a 10 or 11 mm reusable trocar is inserted into the peritoneal cavity. Inspection is carried out with a 0° or a 45° laparoscope.

If unilateral or bilateral indirect hernias are encountered, I use a transperitoneal approach. This involves entering the preperitoneal space by incising the peritoneum and preperitoneal fascia at the orifice of the indirect hernial sac. I prefer this approach, especially for long indirect hernias, as a totally extraperitoneal approach is particularly difficult because the sac is strongly anchored in the inguinal canal. It is difficult to get sufficient space for exposure, and also to dissect the vas and spermatic vessels from the peritoneal sac. Some investigators, however, report no difficulties with a totally extraperitoneal approach, even with indirect hernias[40]. This approach can

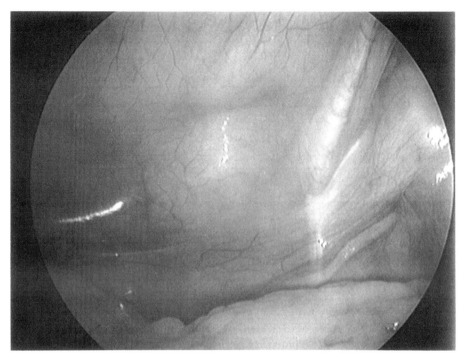

Figure 7.11: On this patient with bilateral direct inguinal hernias, a thickening of the preperitoneal fascia can be seen clearly going from the left (medially) to the right (laterally), along with the vas deferens over the umbilical ligament, and then proceeding anteriorly and laterally to the internal ring which is marked by a small dimple in the peritoneum as well as by the disappearance of the vas deferens.

also be used for direct hernias, although a totally extraperitoneal approach is more easily performed and a peritoneal incision and subsequent closure are avoided along with the theoretical potential for intraperitoneal adhesions. Alternatively, a totally extraperitoneal approach can be accomplished with the open cutdown technique. Once a small cutdown is made in the midline fascia in the infraumbilical area, the preperitoneal space is entered and blunt dissection is carried out with a small finger. The cannula is inserted and further dissection is carried out with the operating laparoscope aided by a blunt dissector introduced through the 5 mm port of the laparoscope (*see* Figure 7.14). Once adequate space has been created, additional ports are placed.

Either with a totally extraperitoneal or a transperitoneal entrance into the preperitoneal and retroperitoneal space, further dissection is carried out with a blunt grasping forceps. Again, care must be taken about being in the correct plane of dissection. The peritoneum and the preperitoneal fascia are easily separated from the posterior inguinal wall medial to the epigastric vessels. Even with direct and recurrent direct hernias the plane is usually easily found, and reduction of the peritoneal sac with associated preperitoneal fascia and preperitoneal fat is easily accomplished. Dissection lateral to the epigastric vessels and especially around the internal ring is somewhat more confusing and complex. The difficulty encountered is due to the often long peritoneal sac, with its accompanying preperitoneal fascia which is usually very adherent to the cord structures both proximal to the orifice of the internal ring and

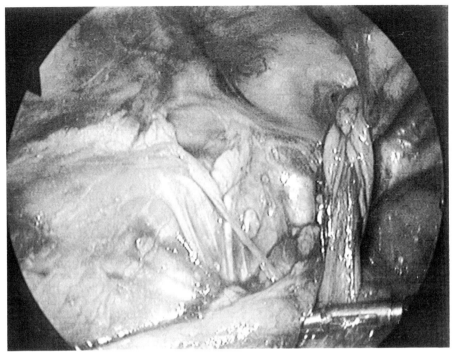

Figure 7.12: Below the iliopubic tract and lateral to the retracted spermatic vessels and cord, the genitofemoral nerve branches can be seen during preperitoneal dissection of this left inguinal hernia.

in the inguinal canal. At the orifice of the internal ring, moreover, when an indirect hernia is present, there is usually a thickening of the peritoneum and preperitoneal fascia, especially medially. This thickening is often associated with a fusion of fibres of the transversalis fascia, the preperitoneal fascia and peritoneum (*see* Figure 7.5). Either with transperitoneal or totally extraperitoneal entry into the preperitoneal space, some sharp dissection may be needed to reduce or transect the sac composed of peritoneum and preperitoneal tissues. Once this is accomplished, lateral dissection can be carried out. Again, dissection of the peritoneum and associated fibrous tissue can be somewhat difficult due to the firm adherence to the cord structures. This dissection can often be aided by transperitoneal visualization, as a 5 mm trocar is inserted into the preperitoneal space for blunt dissection using a blunt grasper and insufflation of carbon dioxide into this space (*see* Figure 7.15). Lateral and proximal dissection should be for at least 4 or 5 cm to allow generous lateral placement of the mesh. After completing the dissection, one should be able to identify the midline, rectus muscle, Cooper's ligament, iliopubic tract, aponeurosis of the transversus abdominis muscle, epigastric vessels, external iliac vein, vas deferens, spermatic vessels, lateral iliopubic tract and origin of the transversus abdominis muscle; and occasionally, below the the iliopubic tract, the genitofemoral nerve can be seen lateral to the spermatic vessels (*see* Figures 7.7 and 7.12). At this point prolene mesh or other material is prepared by trimming the corners for easier manipulation. The mesh should be approximately 10 × 15 cm which will cover Hesselbach's

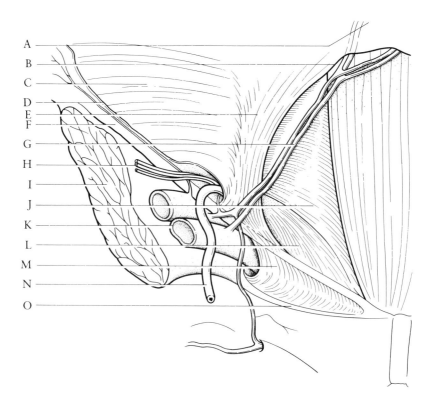

A
B
C
D
E
F
G
H
I
J
K
L
M
N
O

Figure 7.13: Anatomy of the preperitoneal space. (From Lichtenstein IL (1986) Surgical anatomy of the inguinal region. In: Ishiyaku Euroamica Ltd. *Hernia repair without disability*, 2nd ed, with permission.)

triangle, femoral canal, and the internal ring with a minimum 3 cm of margin beyond the limits of the hernia (*see* Figure 7.2).

With large direct hernias, the redundant attenuated transversalis fascia is often loosely approximated with a figure-of-eight or purse-string of 2-0 vicryl suture to flatten the hernia defect and effectively provide a buttress for the mesh which might reduce the chances of the mesh herniating through an open fascial defect (*see* Figure 7.16). With large indirect hernias, if the transversalis fascia sling is sufficiently strong and redundant enough for suture approximation, this defect will be closed (although this is of questionable benefit). Approximation under tension is avoided. In earlier repairs, a minimum of three sutures of 2-0 vicryl were placed on Cooper's ligament or iliopubic tract, aponeurosis of the transversus abdominis muscle, and transversus abdominis and transversalis fascia lateral to the internal ring. This triangle of sutures serves to prevent migration or herniation of the mesh (*see* Figure 7.2). Recently, in part due to the difficulty of suturing and the possibility of edges of the mesh curling which might predispose to reherniation, hernia staples have been used to secure the edges. If the hernia defect is small, sometimes only staples are used. If the hernia defect is large, the mesh is firmly secured with non-absorbable suture with deep bites into strong fascial

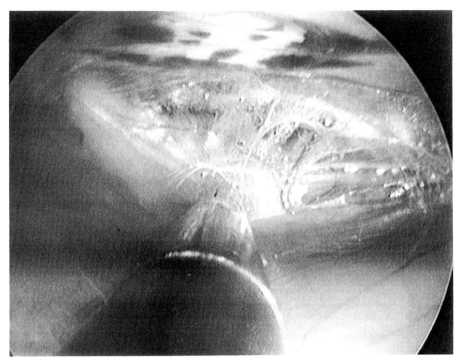

Figure 7.14: The preperitoneal space has been entered through the umbilicus for a totally extraperitoneal dissection. The grasping forceps is being used to dissect.

tissue. The edges are then stapled down to prevent curling of the graft (*see* Figure 7.16D). Initially 2-0 vicryl absorbable suture on a reinforced curved needle was used for ease of handling and the feeling that the mesh would be well absorbed by the time that the vicryl reabsorbed. Recently, however, I have started using Ethibon, silk, Gortex, or other non-absorbable suture. This change was prompted by a recurrence, after a patient was involved in a car accident five weeks after surgery. Three months after the accident he noticed a recurrent bulge in the left inguinal area. I think that the vicryl must have reabsorbed by the time of the accident, and that the impact propelled the abdominal contents onto the large piece of mesh and caused a slippage of the lateral aspect of the mesh from the internal ring, uncovering this area and predisposing to a recurrence. Non-absorbable sutures might have prevented the slippage of this mesh, which might not have been completely incorporated at the time of the accident. Perhaps a more lateral placement or a larger graft could also have prevented this recurrence. More recently, we no longer use any anchoring of mesh.

If a totally extraperitoneal repair is carried out and the patient has a peritoneal hernia sac with a narrow orifice which could predispose to internal herniation, an endoloop is used to close off the sac. If the sac has a wide orifice, however, it is left alone (*see* Figure 7.16E). Any significant tears in the peritoneal lining should be closed to prevent migration and herniation of the intra-abdominal contents into the preperitoneal space. If the repair is performed through an incision in the peritoneum, then the peritoneal defect is closed with a purse-string suture of 3-0 vicryl. Once the peritoneal defects

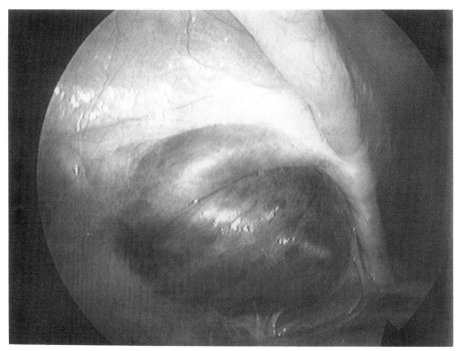

Figure 7.15: Preperitoneal insufflation of carbon dioxide through a lateral port during repair of a left indirect inguinal hernia.

are closed, the carbon dioxide is evacuated with a suction cannula and, during transperitoneal viewing, the mesh is inspected to ensure that it is lying flat (*see* Figure 7.17).

The trocars are then removed and the peritoneal cavity evacuated. The fascial defect from trocar punctures of 10 mm or greater are closed with 2-0 vicryl. The skin incisions are then approximated with subcutaneous 3-0 vicryl sutures. The approximated skin edges are then covered with collodion.

Patients are kept in the recovery room for approximately one hour, then observed for an additional one or two hours in the out-patient holding area. Occasionally patients are admitted for overnight stay. The great majority of patients do not have to observe any weight restrictions; they are allowed to do what they feel comfortable doing, although they should avoid driving for three or four days. Fifteen tablets of hydrocodone 7.5 mg are prescribed. Patients are instructed to take one or two as needed, as frequently as every three hours. The patients are followed up a week postoperatively, and subsequent follow-up is at one month, six months and one year. Long-term follow-up is also planned.

Instrumentation

Most of the procedure can be performed with the instruments that are standard for laparoscopic cholecystectomy. However, dissection and visualization are greatly aided by a 30° or 45° view laparoscope. I particularly favour an Olympus 45° view scope (Olympus Corp., Lake Success, New York). This

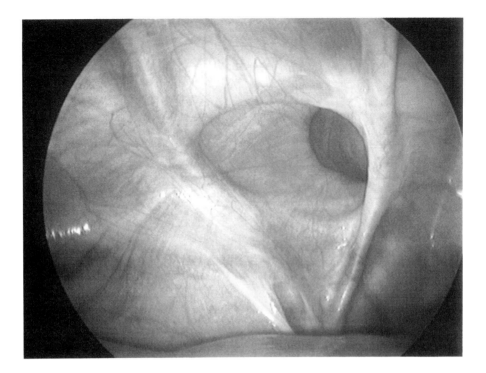

Figure 7.16A: Direct left inguinal hernia.

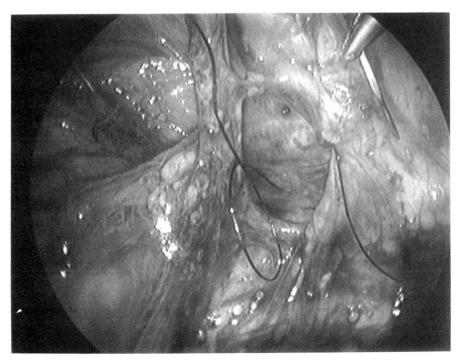

Figure 7.16B: Preperitoneal view of sutures being placed to loosely close the direct defect.

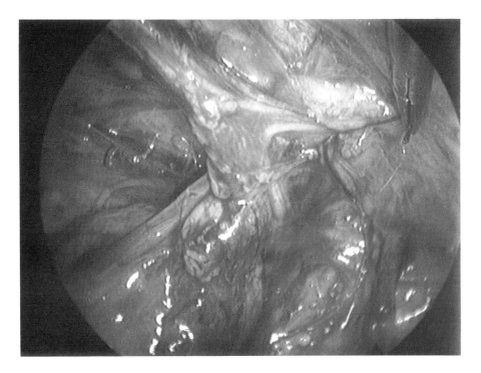

Figure 7.16C: Closed direct defect.

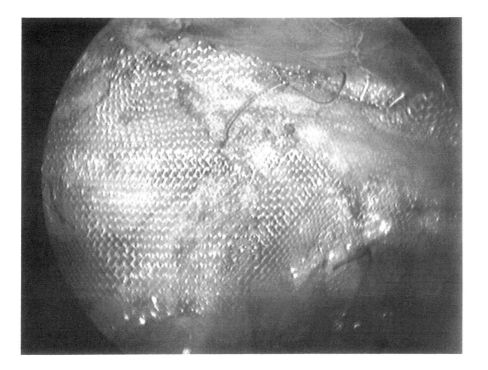

Figure 7.16D: Mesh covering inguinal area and anchored with both sutures and staples.

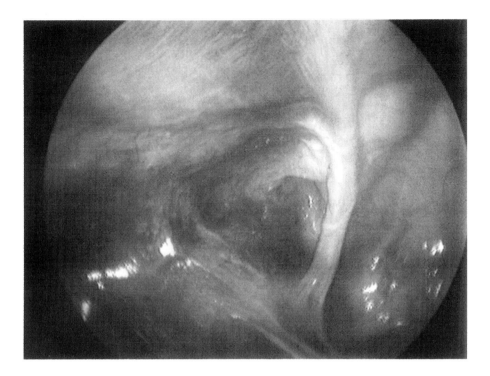

Figure 7.16E: Transperitoneal view of completed extraperitoneal repair.

scope not only provides a greater angle but also seems to have superior light delivery. A 0° laparoscope can be used, but it may be hard to view the anterior abdominal wall when placing sutures or staples. If a totally extraperitoneal dissection is carried out, an operating laparoscope will greatly aid dissection since a blunt dissecting forceps can be inserted through the 5 mm operating channel until adequate space is created to allow insertion of a second trocar in the preperitoneal space.

A proper needle holder is essential. In order to place a suture into Cooper's ligament, a firm grip of a curved needle is necessary. Various needle holders are available, but the two that I most frequently use include the Cook curved needle holder (Cook Ob/gyn, Spencer, Indiana) and an Ethicon needle holder (Ethicon Inc, New Brunswick, New Jersey). The disadvantage with the Cook curved needle holder is that it can only hold the curved needle at a 90° angle to the shaft. If you need to proceed in a 45° anterior or posterior direction, a separate needle holder needs to be substituted. Moreover, it is quite difficult to perform instrument ties with the Cook device. Its advantages are its durability and its ability to hold the needle firmly. However, the Ethicon needle holder has many more advantages. The shaft can be rotated to position the jaw at an optimum angle to the handle. The jaw itself has a diamond pattern tungsten carbide surface which is atraumatic to suture when performing instrument ties. The handle, which comes off the shaft at approximately 45°, has a ratcheted locking mechanism. The disadvantages include a ratchet that is difficult to disengage, and a fragile pin in the centre of the shaft which

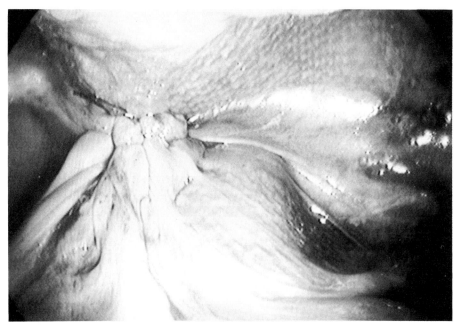

Figure 7.17: View of the peritoneal closure of a transperitoneally repaired indirect right inguinal hernia. The mesh is seen to lie flat.

activates the jaw. This pin mechanism, which is fairly standard, is too fragile for the amount of force required to hold a curved needle firmly. My first needle holder broke at this location. In many circumstances, there is an advantage to a handle in line with the shaft, or at 0° rather than at an angle.

Hernia staplers are now being manufactured by both Ethicon and United States Surgical Corporation. The Ethicon reusable stapler (ES100 Hernia Tacker, Ethicon Inc, Cinncinnati, Ohio) requires a 12 mm trocar for insertion. This is a straight and multiply reloadable single-fire tacker which delivers a staple which is rectangular when closed, resembling the skin staples commonly used in open surgery, and which can attain reasonably deep penetration of tissue. Occasionally this configuration will allow tacking of mesh onto Cooper's ligament, but in my experience the non-deflectable tip makes it hard to obtain the right angle to apply the staple properly. Moreover, the staples are mounted in an unstable manner and fall off easily. This tacker is also available in a multiple-fire disposable version (EMS Rotating Stapler, Ethicon Inc, Cinncinnati, Ohio). Ethicon has also developed a disposable product with a deflectable and rotatable tip (Endopath Endoscopic Articulating Stapler-EAS-60°, Ethicon Inc, Cinncinnati, Ohio) which will probably greatly facilitate staple placement. The United States Surgical Corporation currently has a stapler with a deflectable tip (Endo Hernia Stapler, United States Surgical Corp, Norwalk, Connecticut); it places a staple which looks like a paper staple when closed and which seems to penetrate the tissue less. The most notable disadvantages of any of the disposable staplers is in expense, and the fact that they hold only 10 to 12 staples at a time. They also require 12 mm trocars which could predispose to hernia formation. With these large trocars, consideration should be given to deep closure of these abdominal wall incisions. Alternatively, when the trocar is inserted, an attempt should be made to insert it obliquely so that there will be overlapping of muscle and fascia to cover the various defects at different levels.

Results of laparoscopic preperitoneal mesh repair

In our own series we have performed 105 hernia repairs in 88 patients (86 males and two females; age range 17–83 years) between October 1990 and April 1992. There were 42 left, 34 right and 12 bilateral hernias; 41 were direct, 62 indirect and two femoral, and 15 were recurrent. 87 patients underwent a general anaesthetic and one had an epidural block. 70 had a transabdominal preperitoneal repair, while 35 underwent a totally extraperitoneal repair. There were no intraoperative complications and no conversions to open surgery. Postoperative complications included two inguinal canal haematomas, two case of transient testicular tenderness, one case of transient anterior thigh pain and one umbilical infection. The longest follow-up has been 7.5 months, with an average follow-up of less than two months.

Filipi has now repaired 17 hernias on 16 patients using a transperitoneal approach. He has had one recurrence with a direct hernia. Postoperative complications include one case of difficulty with voiding, two urinary retentions and one lateral thigh discomfort[30].

Barry McKernan, who uses a totally extraperitoneal approach without entering the peritoneal cavity, reports 46 repairs in 34 patients. There have been 27 direct and 19 indirect, with 12 bilateral and 11 recurrent. Postoperative complications include one orchitis and four seromas in large direct hernia defects. He has reported no recurrences yet, but has a short follow-up[40]. Aronoff likewise uses a totally extraperitoneal approach to inguinal hernias. Rather than placing the mesh on top of the cord structures, he makes a slit in the mesh and wraps the mesh around the cord structures for indirect hernias. The mesh he uses is 8 × 4 cm. For direct hernias, a smaller mesh is used over the defect. A combination of suturing and stapling is used. He reports no recurrences in 45 repairs performed since April 1991 on 40 patients. The average follow-up has been nine months. There were five bilateral hernias (10 direct, 30 indirect and five femoral). Postoperative complications include transient scrotal pain in two patients and seromas in 20 % of cases usually associated with repair of large direct defects[41,42].

Gardiner has had a similar experience with a transperitoneal approach to a preperitoneal repair. He has operated on 43 patients to repair 46 hernias. There were 26 direct and 20 indirect hernias. Two were converted to open. He has had no postoperative complications or recurrences[43]. Katkhouda, with the preperitoneal mesh repair, has repaired 73 hernias including four bilateral, seven femoral, 48 direct, 25 indirect, and three recurrent hernias. One conversion to open was required because of hypercapnia during the extraperitoneal approach. Postoperative complications include one scrotal oedema, one with postoperative pain, and one with hypaesthesia of the groin. He has had no recurrence to date with this approach[36]. Begin, in

Dijon, France, has performed 52 laparoscopic preperitoneal hernia repairs (30 direct and 15 indirect) on 45 patients. There have been no operative complications. Postoperatively he has had four haematomas, and there has been one recurrence[44]. Dion has repaired 18 with a preperitoneal mesh (9 × 6 cm) and has had one postoperative complication of testicular pain lasting five days. He has had no recurrences[23,24]. Litwin uses a 9 × 13 cm mesh to cover the inguinal area after filling the hernia defect with small umbrella-shaped pieces of mesh. With this preperitoneal technique, he has repaired 80 hernias with no recurrences[45].

In the collective experience of 11 surgeons whose work has been cited in this chapter, 691 hernias have been repaired by the preperitoneal approach. To date there have been three recurrences (an incidence of 0.43%). However, the follow-up remains too short for any long-term conclusions to be drawn.

Future studies

Laparoscopic herniorrhaphy, as with other laparoscopic procedures, is such a new technique that there are many issues and controversies that need to be resolved. These include the added risk of general anaesthesia and the laparoscopic approach; the added cost of equipment and increased length of the procedure; the routine use of mesh even with simple small indirect defects; the increased potential for intra-abdominal adhesions (especially with use of intraperitoneal mesh, but also with the peritoneal defects which are created and repaired during preperitoneal repairs). Will any of these techniques compare with the successful current approaches and thereby justify the increased risks and costs?

Although many who are performing laparoscopic hernia repairs report a quicker recovery, less pain and a more rapid return to work, many performing open anterior approaches (such as the Shouldice, anterior plug and tensionless patch repairs) report similar rapid recovery times with minimal pain using procedures performed under local anaesthesia as an out-patient. In order to show any advantages, comparisons will need to be made in a prospective manner using a standardized preoperative, operative and postoperative evaluation scheme. Since no single surgeon will be skilled in all the open and laparoscopic approaches, this study cannot be randomized and will probably have to be a multiple institutional study with skilled surgeons performing those particular repairs in which they are proficient. Moreover, this study will probably require several years to complete to determine the long-term recurrence rate. Currently it would probably be premature to start the study, since many techniques are still evolving. There have already been some techniques which have been abandoned; Schultz and Corbitt no longer rely on small mesh plugs, and Fitzgibbons no longer uses intraperitoneal mesh alone for the repair of direct inguinal hernias. Larger meshes are increasingly being used. New techniques tend to be based on previous open procedures (such as the Stoppa and Nyhus preperitoneal repair) but are being performed with different equipment, and using different perspectives.

The changing technology will also play a role in the repair techniques ultimately used. Suturing, stapling and even video imaging are all in their infancy. Perhaps since we are now looking more closely at the various techniques of anterior herniorrrhaphy, and attempting to develop new techniques because of cost considerations and the patient-driven demand for minimal access surgery, we will be given the impetus to develop a more uniform and successful approach to inguinal hernia repair either by the open anterior approach or laparoscopy.

References

1 Polister P and Cunico E (eds) (1989) *Socio-economic factbook for surgery,* American College of Surgeons, Chicago. pp.25–42.

2 Condon RE and Nyhus LM (1989) Complications of groin hernias. In: Nyhus LM, Condon RE (eds) *Hernia.* JB Lippincott, Philadelphia. pp.106–18.

3 Arregui ME *et al.* (1991) Four surgeons describe their separate techniques for performing laparoscopic inguinal hernia repair. *Gen. Surg. News,* 1:23–5.

4 Arregui ME (1992) Laparoscopic hernia repair. *Laparoscopy in Focus,* 1:5.

5 Arregui ME *et al.* (1992) Laparoscopic mesh repair of inguinal hernia using a preperitoneal approach: a preliminary report. *Surg. Laparosc. Endosc.* 2:53–8.

6 Wantz GE (1988) Shouldice repair. *Contemp. Surg.* 33:15–21.

7 Lichtenstein IL (1987) Herniorrhaphy: a personal experience with 6,321 cases. *Amer. J. Surg.* 153:553–9.

8 Gilbert AI (1989) Prosthetic adjuncts to groin hernia repair: a classification of inguinal hernias. *Contemp. Surg.* 32:28–35.

9 Martin RE and Shureih S (1983) The use of marlex mesh in primary hernia repairs. *Surgical Rounds.*

10 Stoppa RE *et al.* (1984) The use of dacron in the repair of hernias of the groin. *Surg. Clin. North Amer.* 64:269–85.

11 Stoppa RE (1989) The treatment of complicated groin and incisional hernias. *World J. Surg.* 13:545–54.

12 Stoppa RE and Warlaumont CR (1989) The preperitoneal approach and prosthetic repair of groin hernia. In: Nyhus LM and Condon RE (eds) *Hernia.* JB Lippincott, Philadelphia. pp.199–225.

13 Nyhus LM *et al.* (1988) The preperitoneal approach and prosthetic buttress repair for recurrent hernia: the evolution of technique. *Ann. Surg.* 208:733–7.

14 Martin RE *et al.* (1982) Polypropylene mesh in 450 hernia repairs: evaluation of wound infections. *Contemp. Surg.* 20:46–8.

15 Nyhus LM (1989) The preperitoneal approach and iliopubic tract repair of inguinal hernia. In: Nyhus LM and Condon RE (eds) *Hernia*. JB Lippincott, Philadelphia. pp.154–88.

16 Ger R (1982) The management of certain abdominal herniae by intra-abdominal closure of the neck of the sac. *Ann. J. R. Coll. Surg. Engl.* **64**:342–4.

17 Ger R *et al.* (1990) Management of indirect inguinal hernias by laparoscopic closure of the neck of the sac. *Am. J. Surg.* **159**:370–3.

18 Ger R (1991) The laparoscopic management of groin hernias. *Contemp. Surg.* **39**:15–19.

19 Ger R (1992) Personal communication.

20 Rosin RD (1992) Personal communication.

21 Spaw AT *et al.* (1991) Laparoscopic hernia repair: the anatomical basis. *J. Laparoendosc. Surg.* **1**:269–77.

22 Spaw AT (1992) Personal communication.

23 Dion YM and Morin J (1992) Laparoscopic inguinal herniorrhaphy. *Can. J. Surg.* **35**:209–12.

24 Dion YM (1992) Personal communication.

25 Shlain L (1992) Personal communication.

26 Franklin M (1992) Laparoscopic hernia repair. *Laparoscopy in Focus.* **1**:7.

27 Franklin M (1992) Personal communication.

28 Salerno GM *et al.* (1991) Laparoscopic inguinal hernia repair. In: Zucker KA (ed.): *Surgical laparoscopy*. Quality Medical Publishing, St. Louis. pp.281–93.

29 Fitzgibbons RJ (1992) *Laparoscopic inguinal herniorrhaphy*. Paper presented at the Society of American Gastrointestinal Endoscopic Surgeons (SAGES) meeting, April 10–12, Washington DC.

30 Filipi CJ (1992) Personal communication.

31 Schultz L *et al.* (1990) Laser laparoscopic herniorrhaphy: a clinical trial. Preliminary results. *J. Laparoendosc. Surg.* **1**:41–5.

32 Corbitt J (1991) Laparoscopic herniorrhaphy. *Surg. Laparosc. Endosc.* **1**:23–5.

33 Schultz L (1992) Personal communication.

34 Schultz L *et al.* (1992) *Laparoscopic inguinal herniorrhaphy – lessons learned after 100 cases*. Video presentation, Society of Gastrointestinal Endoscopic Surgeons (SAGES), April 10–12, Washington DC.

35 Corbitt J (1992) Laparoscopic hernia repair. *Laparoscopy in Focus*. 1:4.

36 Katkhouda N (1992) Personal communication.

37 Schafmayer A *et al.* (1992) Personal communication.

38 MacFadyen BV (1992) *Complications of laparoscopic inguinal hernia repair.* Paper presented at the Society of American Gastrointestinal Endoscopic Surgeons (SAGES) meeting, April 10–12, Washington DC.

39 Anson BJ *et al.* (1960) Surgical anatomy of the inguinal region based upon a study of 500 body halves. *Surg. Gyn. Obst.* 111:707–25.

40 McKernan JB (1992) Personal communication.

41 Aronhoff RJ (1992*a*) Laparoscopic hernia repair. *Laparoscopy in Focus*. 1:5–7.

42 Aronhoff RJ (1992*b*) Personal communications.

43 Gardiner B (1992) Personal communication.

44 Begin GF (1992) Personal communication.

45 Litwin D (1992) Personal communication.

8

Laparoscopic Common Duct Exploration

JOSEPH B. PETELIN

Since laparoscopic cholecystectomy was introduced in 1986[1], thousands of surgeons have learned the basic technique of the operation. The surgeon with relatively little experience with laparoscopic cholecystectomy may choose patients in whom he suspects there is little chance of common duct pathology, and in whom he selectively omits cholangiography. As he becomes more skilled, however, he may broaden the indications for this less invasive technique and is likely to encounter patients with choledocholithiasis. Such an evolution in technical competence is only natural, and it should stimulate an equally natural evolution in the scope of treatment possibilities for patients with biliary tract disease. Certainly most surgeons agree, that if laparoscopic gallbladder surgery is to stand the test of time, all aspects of surgical biliary tract disease must be handled at least as effectively as they are in 'open' surgery.

Laparoscopic treatment of choledocholithiasis represents the next logical subject that the general surgeon should master in his quest to treat all aspects of gallstone disease in a minimal access fashion. Interestingly, critics of laparoscopic cholecystectomy initially suggested that this would be impossible because the porta hepatis would be very poorly visualized during laparoscopic surgery. Intraoperative cholangiograms were thought to be 'nearly impossible' to obtain and, for this reason, many felt they would not be employed as frequently as they would have been under open surgery. The thought of exploring the common bile duct under laparoscopic guidance seemed like sheer madness. Nevertheless, all of these preconceived notions have been dispelled. The view of the porta hepatis is not only comparable to that obtained in open surgery: it is in fact much superior, owing of course to the magnification afforded by the scopes and camera systems. This has allowed the development of techniques whereby intraoperative cholangiograms may be routinely performed without difficulty. Many surgeons feel that laparoscopic cholangiography is actually easier to perform than its open counterpart[2,3].

Laparoscopic common duct exploration, however, has not yet been widely practised. This is understandable, since it requires more sophisticated equipment and considerably more skill on the part of the surgeon. This slow and cautious movement of surgical attention and intervention, from the gallbladder toward the common duct, parallels the history of open biliary tract surgery. Indeed, although the first cholecystectomy was performed by Langenbuch in July 1882, the first successful common duct exploration was not performed until January 1890 by Courvoisier[4]. Fortunately, the ability to explore the common duct laparoscopically did not take eight years to develop; it has already been effectively employed in hundreds of cases, albeit by relatively few surgeons.

This chapter will explore the techniques and technology currently available for laparoscopic treatment of common duct problems. Even as this material is being published, however, new developments may already have rendered some of these ground-breaking concepts and technologies obsolete. The reader is encouraged to entertain these ideas with the same perspective that an explorer or an inventor might use, and to regard this chapter as a 'guide' rather than a 'bible' in the surgical approach to common duct pathology.

Preoperative evaluation and patient selection

The histories given by patients with choledocholithiasis are often similar to those given by patients with uncomplicated cholelithiasis or cholecystitis. Common symptoms are right upper-quadrant pain, with or without radiation to the interscapular region, nausea with or without emesis, fever and anorexia. In other cases, more classic symptoms including fever, chills and jaundice suggest ascending cholangitis. Some patients present with signs and symptoms of biliary pancreatitis.

Examination usually reveals right upper-quadrant tenderness. Rarely, the distended gallbladder may be palpated. Jaundice may or may not be apparent clinically, and the urine may or may not be dark. No other striking physical findings distinguish the patient with choledocholithiasis from a patient with cholethiasis.

Laboratory and radiological data are usually extremely helpful in making the diagnosis[5], or at least in raising the strong suspicion of the presence of common duct stones. Elevated levels of transaminases, alkaline phosphatase and bilirubin are usually present. In patients with biliary pancreatitis, increased levels of amylase and lipase are usually seen. The white blood count is also usually elevated. Sonogram of the abdomen demonstrates dilatation of the common ductal system in most patients. Very occasionally, sonography confirms the presence of stones in the common duct. Radionuclide studies usually show abnormalities in appearance of the material in the gallbladder, the ductal system and the duodenum. Computed tomography (CT) scans usually reveal dilatation of the ducts, but may or may not disclose the presence of stones. Endoscopic retrograde cholangiopancreatography (ERCP) usually demonstrates the reason for the obstruction and the number of stones present.

Most patients are selected as surgical candidates based on the demonstration of symptomatic gallbladder disease and on their ability to withstand a general anaesthetic. One of two situations will then apply. Either the patient will not be suspected to harbour common duct stones and they will subsequently be found on intraoperative cholangiography; or the preoperative findings will be highly suggestive of choledocholithiasis.

In the first case, the surgeon has a relatively easy decision to make. He may proceed with laparoscopic common duct exploration, convert the operation to an open common duct exploration, or leave the stone(s) in place for subsequent treatment with ERCP, lithotripsy, dissolution, or a combination of the three. These options are usually discussed with the patient preoperatively. Open common duct exploration, laparoscopy and ERCP are all successful in clearing the common duct in over 90% of cases[6]. Clinical data for extracorporeal lithotripsy and dissolution success rates in clearing the ductal system are rare. Likewise, the long-term effects of endoscopic sphincterotomy are not clear. Surgeons question the likelihood of subsequent stricture formation or ascending cholangitis following ERCP. There is a dearth of clinical data regarding this matter, so the surgeon is usually left to make a decision based on his own clinical experience.

In the second case, the surgeon must decide whether to subject the patient to preoperative ERCP, lithotripsy or dissolution therapy. While the latter two choices are relatively easy to pass over, the decision to proceed with preoperative ERCP is more difficult. Early in one's experience with laparoscopic biliary tract surgery, it is often wise to consider preoperative ERCP when there is a high likelihood of common duct stones. Conventional wisdom has suggested that this choice is easiest in patients over 60 years of age, since they do not have to live with the potentially negative side effects of ERCP for as long as a 30-year-old might. This approach certainly seems most sensible in the more frail elderly individual. Its application in younger patients is more controversial, and until there are enough data to judge each approach, the surgeon is compelled to use his best judgement. This should obviously be based on his experience and on the patient's clinical presentation.

In either case, the surgeon will be required to balance the positive effects of minimal access surgery against the potential need for subsequent intervention, such as ERCP or even second stage open common duct exploration, each with its own morbidity. The reader should be able to construct his own algorithm regarding his approach to common duct stones, but a suggested protocol is presented in Figure 8.1. As the surgeon becomes more adept at laparoscopic surgery, he should find it easier to solve common duct problems. Certainly, his willingness to select laparoscopic common duct exploration over ERCP will approach the same level as it occupied for 'open' surgery.

Indications for laparoscopic common duct exploration may include jaundice, abnormal liver function tests suggesting possible common duct pathology, an abnormally dilated common duct identified on sonography or CT scan, an abnormal radionuclide scan, recent history of biliary pancreatitis, history suggestive of cholangitis, and abnormal intraoperative cholangiogram, 'palpable' common duct stones (ballottable), or high index of suspicion of ductal pathology. Of these possible indications, intraoperative cholangiography is

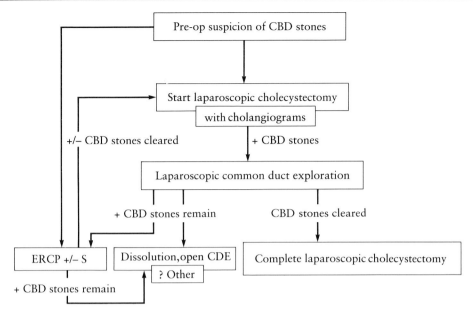

Figure 8.1: A protocol for common duct stones.

the most likely to present evidence supporting the need for common duct exploration.

Intraoperative cholangiography

Discussion of the treatment of choledocholithiasis must include cholangiography. During the past decade, a movement away from routine cholangiography to a selective approach has been advocated[7,8]. While there may be sound arguments for this stance in open surgery, new considerations in laparoscopic biliary tract surgery make such a position less attractive.

First of all, since laparoscopic cholecystectomy is still a relatively new procedure, most surgeons have little experience of its various manoeuvres. The surgeon would be wise to 'practise' at first, performing *routine* cholangiography during laparoscopic cholecystectomy until he is confident that he could perform it in any circumstances.

Secondly, since the anatomy is usually viewed from the umbilicus in laparoscopic surgery, the relationship between the ductal structures may be more difficult to appreciate than it is in open surgery. Cholangiography allows another perspective and gives precise radiographic delineation of the ductal anatomy, especially in those cases where severe inflammatory changes or ductal anomalies make identification of the branches of the extrahepatic biliary tree essential to the safe conduct of the operation.

Thirdly, since there has been a tendency to leave a longer cystic duct remnant when cholecystectomy is performed laparoscopically, it is imperative to ensure that no stones are left in the remnant so that subsequent choledocholithiasis does not occur. Finally, evaluation of the common ductal system for stones deserves the same consideration as in open surgery.

Once the surgeon is comfortable with his ability to perform laparoscopic cholangiograms and to interpret the anatomy from the new perspective, then a selective approach to intraoperative cholangiography may be appropriate. (The author and a number of other accomplished laparoscopic biliary tract surgeons, however, prefer routine cholangiography even after these conditions have been met.) Until the surgeon has gained considerable experience, laparoscopic cholangiography should be routinely attempted so long as such activity does not interfere with the welfare of the patient. A logical approach would involve allocation of five or ten minutes per case for cystic duct cannulation early in one's experience with laparoscopic cholecystectomy. If in that period of time the surgeon is unsuccessful, and if there is little likelihood of common duct stones, then selective abandonment of the attempt should be considered. This assumes of course, that the surgeon is absolutely sure of the ductal anatomy and of the fact that there are no stones in the cystic duct remnant.

Two basic techniques have evolved. In the *port access* technique, the cystic duct is cannulated with a standard cholangiographic catheter which is inserted through one of the 5 mm ports already in place in the right upper quadrant. This technique was first employed by Reddick and Olsen[9], and required the use of a specially designed clamp, which not only guided the catheter into the cystic duct but also fixed it into position. This device is inserted either through the most lateral port or the mid-clavicular port, depending on the surgeon's preference. It has the advantage of allowing placement and fixation with the same instrument. It does, however, have several disadvantages.

First of all, since one of the ports is used for access, exposure in the porta hepatis is often compromised, even after the grasping forceps in the other port is 'adjusted' (an extra step). Secondly, since the forceps is often inserted from the right side of table, an experienced assistant is usually required on that side of table (unless the surgeon goes to the right side of the table and inserts the device himself. Once he is experienced, he may be able to insert it while remaining on the left side of the patient.) Thirdly, the insertion instrument is not inexpensive. Finally, since the device is radio-opaque, it must be oriented so as not to obscure the ductal system on the radiograph.

Newer devices have been developed since this ground-breaking technique was established, and the reader is advised to research local availability of these inventions in this ever-expanding armamentarium.

The *percutaneous* technique of cholangiography, developed by Petelin in January 1990, involves placement of a standard cholangiocatheter into the cystic duct via a percutaneous sleeve. The sleeve, a standard 14 gauge polyethylene IV catheter, is inserted through the abdominal wall in a cephalad direction. It is located approximately 2–3 cm medial to the mid-clavicular port. The cholangiocatheter is then inserted through this sleeve, grasped with forceps inserted through the medial epigastric port, and directed into the cystic duct. It is fixed into position with a standard metal clip partially applied across the catheter and duct. This arrangement allows a watertight seal and adequate flow of contrast into the ductal system. Newer catheters, which feature balloon fixation devices incorporated into the catheter itself, are preferred by some surgeons, although they are much more expensive than the older standard catheters.

The percutaneous technique has several advantages over the portal technique. First of all, exposure is maintained, since none of the grasping forceps used to control the gallbladder is removed. Secondly, no expensive device is required to fix the catheter in place. Thirdly, the materials are radiolucent, thereby avoiding radiographic problems. Finally, the sleeve may be subsequently used to insert Fogarty balloon catheters during common duct exploration. If the cholangiograms are normal, the catheter is easily removed from the duct, and the sleeve is sealed with a standard cap until the procedure is completed.

Both techniques of cholangiography have merit. The surgeon should familiarize himself with at least one of them and become proficient in its application.

Equipment required for laparoscopic common duct exploration

In addition to the basic equipment necessary to perform laparoscopic cholecystectomy, a limited number of instruments are required to facilitate common duct exploration[10,11].

Fogarty embolectomy catheters can be very useful during laparoscopic common duct exploration. In this setting, the standard vascular type of catheter is preferred, since the biliary Fogarty catheter is not long enough. Although a 4 French size is most commonly used, 3 French and 5 French models may occasionally be useful. The 4 French catheter fits snugly into the 14 gauge percutaneous sleeve used for cholangiography (*see* p. 275).

A flexible choledochoscope is absolutely essential in order to perform laparoscopic common duct exploration in most cases. Older models which exceeded 5 mm in outside diameter are not useful here. The most versatile scopes now feature a maximum outside diameter of approximately 3 mm, deflection in at least one direction, a working channel of 1 mm and excellent optics. A number of models are currently available.

The flexible scope requires a separate light source with automatic iris capabilities. Although the scope may be used under direct visualization by the surgeon, its manipulation is facilitated by application of a second camera system to its eyepiece. This allows the surgeon the use of both hands during manipulation. Since the image is projected onto the video screen, the other members of the team may be able to assist more effectively. This does, however, require an additional video monitor for viewing.

Alternatively, a video-mixing system (Figure 8.2) may be used to produce a picture-in-picture effect, whereby the choledochoscopic image is projected onto the same monitor as the laparoscopic image. This second image is reduced in size and positioned with a joystick so that it does not interfere with the laparoscopic image. The author has found this system to be the most efficient: it does not produce more clutter in the operating theatre, and the surgeon may view everything on the same monitor instead of transferring his gaze from one to the other. Although the video mixer is currently a separate piece of equipment, a number of manufacturers have been asked to consider incorporating the electronics necessary for mixing into a specifically designed dual-source camera unit. This would allow the cameras from the laparoscope and the choledochoscope to be attached to the same processing unit, light source and monitor.

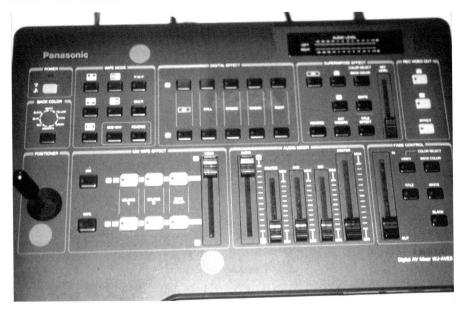

Figure 8.2: A video-mixing system.

Stone retrieval baskets are available in a variety of sizes and configurations, and the surgeon may choose according to his needs. The author finds a 1 mm diameter 4-wire straight basket most useful, but other surgeons have other preferences which work equally well.

Lithotripters may be useful to dissolve large stones in the ductal system. Both electrohydraulic and laser models are available, although the latter are currently prohibitively expensive. Wires or fibres used to deliver the energy to the surface of the stone may be advanced through the working channel of the choledochoscope to the site of the stone.

In most cases, common duct exploration may be performed through the cystic duct[12]. This usually requires dilatation to approximately 12 French size. This may be accomplished with graduated ureteral dilators which are advanced over a guide-wire into the ductal system, or with radial balloon dilators similarly inserted.

In cases where choledochotomy is necessary to allow insertion of the scope, a long-handled scalpel or laser fibre with a contact scalpel is necessary to open the duct[13]. A standard T-tube may be inserted and the choledochotomy closed laparoscopically, but this requires an 8 or 9 mm introduction sleeve to allow placement of the T-tube into the peritoneal cavity. Laparoscopic needle holders are required to allow placement of the sutures necessary to close the common duct.

A 19 French fluted closed suction drain is preferred for drainage of the operative site, although others may also be used effectively.

Operative technique

Overview

Laparoscopic common duct exploration may be accomplished by a single surgeon and a single scrub nurse, who just need a bit more time and stamina to prepare the choledochoscopic equipment. Often the actual ductal exploration requires a rather limited amount of time. Preoperative preparation can minimize the length of the procedure in most cases, although where choledochotomy is necessary the entire procedure will inevitably take significantly more time than uncomplicated laparoscopic cholecystectomy. The surgeon and his team must be physically, emotionally and mentally prepared for this situation: otherwise both decision-making and performance will deteriorate to the extent that laparoscopic ductal exploration will become difficult if not dangerous.

Laparoscopic common duct exploration may be artificially divided into the following stages:

- dissection of the triangle of Calot
- initial manoeuvres to clear the duct
- preparation and placement of the equipment
- dilatation of the cystic duct or choledochotomy
- insertion and manipulation of the scope
- insertion of the basket and entrapment of the stone(s)
- lithotripsy if necessary
- placement of the T-tube/closure of the common duct.

At each stage, specific manoeuvres and precautions facilitate completion in an expeditious manner with the least likelihood for mishap.

Dissection of the triangle of Calot

After all the ports necessary for laparoscopic cholecystectomy have been placed, and after the gallbladder has been retracted, initial dissection of the cystic artery and cystic duct is commenced. Cholangiograms are then obtained by one of the methods previously described. If the cholangiograms are abnormal, then further dissection in the triangle of Calot is usually necessary to delineate the cystic duct–common duct junction adequately and to allow direct access to the common duct. This more thorough dissection is most commonly avoided in laparoscopic cholecystectomy for uncomplicated cholelithiasis and cholecystitis in order to minimize the chances for ductal injury in the routine case.

When it becomes necessary to explore the common bile duct, however, this area must be as clearly defined as possible. As dissection proceeds from the neck of the gallbladder toward the common duct, a variety of manoeuvres may improve exposure.

Patient positioning is often overlooked as an aid in this situation. If the porta hepatis is not well displayed, as is often the case in the obese individual, a reverse Trendelenburg position usually helps. If this is not adequate, then rotation to a slight left lateral decubitus position might be tried. If exposure is still not optimum, it is important to scan the right upper quadrant to ensure that adhesions are not causing the hepatic flexure of the colon to be trapped immediately beneath the liver. A few minutes spent on adhesiolysis in this case will often be repaid with a dramatic improvement in visualization.

Likewise, the duodenal bulb may be inadvertently displaced laterally by a nasogastric tube which has been inserted too far into the stomach. Simple withdrawal will solve this problem easily. It is obviously helpful to have identified the cystic artery already. If it can be clearly delineated from the other structures in this area, such as the right hepatic artery and the cystic duct, it is occasionally useful to clip or ligate it and divide it at this time. This simple step allows the common duct to retract back toward the midline while tension is maintained on the neck of the gallbladder laterally.

Display of the common duct for confirmation of its orientation is often temporarily achieved during its dissection, by using forceps in the medial epigastric port to displace the duodenal bulb inferiorly. This gently stretches the common duct into a taut band which can be identified easily as it extends from the liver to the duodenum. This is only a temporary manoeuvre, but the author has found it extremely useful to confirm the relative positions of the various structures in the porta hepatis.

During more 'medial' dissection it is wise to avoid excessive tension on the neck of the gallbladder, since this may lead to avulsion of the cystic duct; this makes common duct exploration via the cystic duct very difficult.

Initial manoeuvres to clear the duct

When cholangiograms are abnormal, a variety of manoeuvres may be used to clear the the duct. In some cases, no definite stones are found in the duct, but contrast fails to enter the duodenum. Intravenous glucagon, 1 mg IV may be administered to relax the sphincter of Oddi, and the cholangiograms may be attempted again. If this fails, then a 4 French catheter (standard vascular type) may be inserted through the same 14 gauge plastic sleeve used to obtain cholangiograms.

This balloon-tipped catheter may be inserted via the cystic duct into the common duct, and often even into the duodenum. Its location in the duodenum may be verified by inflating the balloon and gradually withdrawing the catheter until it meets resistance at the sphincter. The balloon is then deflated, the catheter is withdrawn another 1 cm, and the balloon is re-inflated if gentle dilatation of the sphincter is desired. The catheter may be further withdrawn from the ductal system, and occasionally the operator is rewarded with the retrieval of the debris occluding the duct. This must be done very gently to avoid damage to the sphincter, postoperative stricture and pancreatitis. These steps are usually accomplished while the nursing team prepares the choledochoscope and its associated equipment for more thorough ductal exploration.

Preparation and placement of equipment

In order to visualize the ductal system thoroughly, and to correct any problems, a flexible fibreoptic choledochoscope is essential. Within the past few years a number of models have been developed. Most of them require significant preparation before use. Since most models are reusable, they have to be sterilized – using either gas (ethylene oxide) or immersion techniques. Since most immersion methods require at least 20 minutes, it is wise to accomplish this before the case starts if there is a high suspicion of choledocholithiasis preoperatively.

Once the scope is prepared, it is brought to the field where it is connected to the light source, irrigation tubing and camera equipment (if available). Proper location of the 'head' of the instrument is a matter of surgeon preference, although the author currently favours placement on a small tray located above the patient's chest. This allows the light-source cable and irrigation tubing to exit the sterile field in a minimally obstructive path. Sterile saline is generally used as the irrigant for the scope. An auto-irising light source presents the most uniform lighting conditions for ductal viewing.

Although a camera is not absolutely necessary for adequate exploration, its application to the choledochoscope greatly enhances the performance of the procedure. The surgeon can then use both hands to manipulate the flexible tip and basket devices to extract stones; otherwise he must hold the head of the scope so that he can view through the eyepiece, which severely limits his ability to manipulate the distal end of the scope and its accessories.

The camera may be attached to another TV monitor, but this usually requires the introduction of another cabinet into the operating room, which may cause considerable crowding. The alternative is for the camera of the choledochoscope, as well as the camera of the laparoscope, to be attached to an audio-video mixer, which incorporates a picture-in-picture effect into its structure. With this system, both images may be projected onto the same TV monitor. Obvious advantages of this configuration include:

- less crowding in the operating room
- better control of the projected images, both being processed by the same mixer
- more efficient visualization of both the laparoscopic and the choledocho-scopic images, since they are both on the same screen.

Dilatation of the cystic duct or choledochotomy

In most cases, laparoscopic common duct exploration may be accomplished through the cystic duct. The duct must be dilated to at least 10 French diameter (approximately 3.3 mm) to allow insertion and/or manipulation of the flexible scope and its accessories. Occasionally, the cystic duct is already large enough to accept the scope; if not, dilatation is necessary, with either graduated or pneumatic dilators.

In both methods, a guide-wire is first inserted through the cystic duct into the common duct. The guide-wire enters the abdominal cavity through the mid-clavicular port. The grasping forceps, which have been controlling the neck of the gallbladder through this port, must be removed first. If this causes problems with exposure, then the forceps in the most lateral port may be moved from the fundus to the neck of the gallbladder, which is then displaced in a cephalad direction. Surprisingly, this step usually results in dramatic improvement in exposure of the triangle of Calot. Once the guide-wire is in place, then the dilator of choice is inserted over it into the ductal system. Once the duct is sufficiently dilated, both the dilators and the guide-wire are removed and the scope is inserted. Alternatively, the guide-wire may be left in place until the scope is advanced over it into the duct.

If the cystic duct is less than 1.5 mm in diameter before manipulation, however, or if it is densely scarred, then it will most likely *not* be able to be enlarged to adequate size to allow introduction of the scope. In this case, the surgeon must decide whether to proceed with laparoscopic choledochotomy, convert to open common duct exploration, or simply complete the laparoscopic cholecystectomy, leaving the stones in the common duct for subsequent postoperative ERC/sphincterotomy. If the first option is chosen, the common duct is opened longitudinally as in open surgery, with a knife, laser or scissors. The surgeon should be cautioned here to limit the length of the choledochotomy to 1 cm or the diameter of the largest stone, whichever is greater; this allows for easy stone removal from the duct, minimal difficulty with T-tube placement, and subsequent closure of a rather small defect in the common duct.

Approaching ductal exploration through a choledochotomy rather than through the cystic duct, offers the added advantage of easier access to the proximal extrahepatic and intrahepatic ductal system, since the flexible scope is much easier to advance in that direction through an opening in the common duct than it is via the cystic duct.

Insertion and manipulation of the scope

Once access to the common duct has been obtained, the scope is inserted through the mid-clavicular port and guided to either the cystic duct access site or the choledochotomy with forceps inserted through the medial–epigastric port. If exposure becomes a problem when the mid-clavicular port is used for the scope, and if replacement of the more lateral forceps from the fundus to the neck of the gallbladder does not improve the situation, then a fifth port, 5 mm in diameter, may be placed in the right upper quadrant to facilitate scope insertion. Although the exact location of this port may vary from case to case, the author finds that a site approximately 7 cm inferior to the mid-clavicular port works quite well.

Once the flexible distal tip of the scope is placed at least 3–4 cm into the duct, the forceps used to aid in its insertion may be temporarily withdrawn from the medial–epigastric port. The surgeon then uses both hands to manipulate the scope. The author usually prefers to use the left hand to control the scope at the level of its insertion into the mid-clavicular port. Actually, only the index finger and thumb of the left hand are used to torque the scope very gently at this level. Meanwhile, the right hand controls the head of the scope with its deflection lever and irrigation port. It is important to note here that constant drip irrigation with normal saline is employed both to dilate the duct and to clear the field of view.

With these manoeuvres, the duct may be negotiated with minimal difficulty. A Kocher manoeuvre is usually not necessary when the flexible scope is used to explore the distal duct. Manipulation of the scope into the proximal ductal system, however, is usually only possible with the current scope technology through a choledochotomy; the cystic duct–common duct junction will rarely be oriented so as to allow retroflexion into the common hepatic duct from the cystic duct. Herein lies a limitation of laparoscopic common duct exploration via the cystic duct. If proximal pathology is suspected, then the surgeon must consider the options previously discussed regarding choledochotomy.

Insertion of the basket and entrapment of the stone(s) with lithotripsy if necessary

The ultimate test of laparoscopic common duct exploration demands clearance of the duct. In most cases, this will require insertion and manipulation of basket(s) to entrap and remove the stones and/or debris. In the author's opinion, this is the most difficult manoeuvre involved in laparoscopic common duct exploration. Firstly, the scope must be properly positioned so that the stones are visible in the duct. Saline is irrigated through the working channel of the scope to allow for distension of the ductal system. Without this irrigation, visualization is nearly impossible.

Once the stones are identified, however, the basket must be inserted through this channel. This significantly impedes any flow of saline into the duct, resulting in limited ability to see and manoeuvre for extended periods of time. Therefore, basketing techniques must be performed expeditiously and precisely. Herein lies the art of laparoscopic common duct exploration.

Commonly, the surgeon must not only manipulate the head of the scope to deflect the distal tip, but must also torque the scope into position in the centre of the duct, while advancing the basket to the stone. He must then open and manipulate the basket around the stone, trap it, and extract the entire ensemble from the duct. Insertion of the basket beyond the stone(s), with subsequent retraction while closing the wires is often the most helpful manoeuvre. Gentle forward and backward movement of the basket in small increments (jiggling) is also very effective in trapping stone(s).

Occasionally, when stones of large size are brought to the cystic–common duct junction, the cystic duct appears to be too small to allow entry of the stone. In these cases, the stone may be crushed with external pressure applied by forceps around the duct, or the cystic duct may be opened longitudinally down onto the common duct until the stone is delivered. Alternatively, intraluminal lithotripsy with laser, electro–hydraulic or mechanical devices may be used to reduce the size of the fragments to a size amenable to removal.

Placement of the T-tube/closure of the common duct

When a choledochotomy has been used to gain access to the common duct, it is usually closed over a T-tube. On first pass, this may seem almost impossible. However, with a little practice in laparoscopic suturing techniques, and with the magnification afforded by the laparoscope and camera system, the surgeon will soon realize that closure of the choledochotomy can actually be done more precisely and with less manipulation than in open surgery.

The T-tube is inserted through the medial epigastric 10 mm port, using an 8 or 9 mm hollow loading tube to facilitate its entry into the peritoneal cavity. The entire tube is placed within the abdomen, and only after it is fixed into position is the catheter advanced out of the peritoneal cavity via the most lateral port. The 'T' portion of the tube is inserted into the duct in a standard fashion. The edges of the duct are then closed with interrupted or continuous suture of 4–0 or 5–0 Vicryl. If interrupted sutures are used, usually only three or four sutures are needed to achieve a water-tight closure. Once the tube is in place and has been fixed outside the abdominal cavity, completion cholangiography is performed. (If the common duct has been explored via the cystic duct, completion cholangiography is performed in standard fashion via the cystic duct.)

Completion of the cholecystectomy

Once the duct has been cleared, the gallbladder is routinely dissected from the liver and removed from the abdomen. It is often wise, in these cases to leave a closed-system drain in place, especially in cases where a choledochotomy has been used. Drain placement is discussed in Chapter 4.

References

1   Muhe E (1986) Die erste Cholezystektomie durch das Laparoskop. *Langenb. Arch. Klin. Chir.* **369**: 804.

2   Appel S, Krebs H and Fern D (1992) Techniques for laparoscopic cholangiography and removal of common duct stones. *Surg. Endosc.* **6**: 134–7.

3   Birkett D (1992) Technique of cholangiography and cystic-duct choledochoscopy at the time of laparoscopic cholecystectomy for laser lithotripsy. *Surg. Endosc.* **6**: 252–4.

4   Beal J (1984) Historical perspective of gallstone disease. *S.G.O.* **158**:181–9.

5   Del Santa P, Kazarian K, Rogers F, Bevins P and Hall J (1985) Prediction of operative cholangiography in patients undergoing elective cholecystectomy with routine liver function chemistries. *Surgery.* **98**: 7–11.

6   Cotton PB (1984) Endoscopic management of bile duct stones (apples and oranges). *Gut.* **25**: 587–97.

7   Grogono JL and Woods W (1986) Selective use of operative cholangiography. *World J. Surg.* **10**: 1009–13.

8   Gregg R (1988) The case for selective cholangiography. *Am. J. Surg.* **155**: 540–5.

9   Reddick EJ, Olsen DO, Daniel JF, Saye WB, McKernan B, Miller W and Hoback M (1989) Laparoscopic laser cholecystectomy. *Laser Med. Surg. News Adv.* 38–40.

10   Hunter J (1992) Laparoscopic transcystic common bile duct exploration. *Am. J. Surg.* **163**: 53–8.

11   Petelin J (1993) Laparoscopic approach to common duct pathology. *Am. J. Surg.* **165**: 487–91.

12   Sackier JM, Berci G and Pas-Partlow M (1991) Laparoscopic transcystic choledochotomy as an adjunct to laparoscopic cholecystectomy. *Amer. Surg.* **57**: 323–6.

13   Jacobs M, Cerdeja JC and Goldstein HS (1991) Laparoscopic choledocholithotomy. *J. Laparoendosc. Surg.* **1**: 79–82.

Suggested further reading

Arregui M, Davis CJ, Arkush AM and Nagan RF (1992) Laparoscopic cholecystectomy combined with endoscopic sphincterotomy and stone extraction or laparoscopic choledochoscopy and electrohydraulic lithotripsy for management of cholelithiasis with choledocholithiasis. *Surg. Endosc.* **6**: 10–15.

Carr-Locke DL (1990) Acute gallstone pancreatitis and endoscopic therapy. *Endosc.* **22**: 180–3.

Carroll BJ, Phillips EH, Daykhovsky L, Grundfest WS, Gersham A, Fallas M and Chandra M (1992) Laparoscopic choledochoscopy: an effective approach to the common duct. *J. Laparoendosc. Surg.* **2**: 15–21.

Dion YM, Morin J, Dionne G and Dejoie C (1992) Laparoscopic cholecystectomy and choledocholithiasis. *C.J.S.* **35**: 67–74.

Fletcher D, Jones RM, O'Riordan B and Hardy KJ (1992) Laparoscopic cholecystectomy for complicated gallstone disease. *Surg. Endosc.* **6**: 179–82.

Petelin J (1990) The argument for contact laser laparoscopic cholecystectomy. *Clin. Laser Monthly.* 71–4.

Petelin J (1991) Laparoscopic approach to common duct pathology. *Surg. Lap. Endosc.* **1**: 33–41.

Petelin J (1993) Clinical results of common bile duct exploration. *Endosc. Surg. Allied Tech.* In press.

Quattlebaum JK and Flanders HD (1991) Laparoscopic treatment of common bile duct stones. *Surg. Lapar. Endosc.* **1**: 26–32.

Reddick EJ and Olsen DO (1990) Personal communication.

Vitale GC, Larson GM, Wieman TJ, Cheadle WG and Miller FB (1993) The use of ERCP in the management of common bile duct stones in patients undergoing laparoscopic cholecystectomy. *Surg. Endosc.* **7**: 9–11.

9

Laparoscopic Nissen Fundoplication

BERNARD DALLEMAGNE

Gastro-oesophageal reflux is a common disease that accounts for approximately 75% of the pathology of the oesophagus[1]. It is often considered synonymous with hiatal hernia, but it is not: reflux can occur in the absence of hiatal hernia, and hernias are often symptom-free[2].

The symptoms of gastro-oesophageal reflux disease (GERD) are classically heartburn or acid regurgitation. They are not specific and can be related to other diseases such as duodenal ulcer, gallstones and other oesophageal disorders. Others symptoms included pseudocardiac pain, vomiting, belching and coughing.

GERD, or increased oesophageal exposure to gastric juice, can be caused by an absence of the lower oesophageal sphincter (LES), an inefficient oesophageal clearance of refluxed gastric juice or an abnormality of the gastric reservoir that augments physiological reflux[1–5]. Hiatal hernia can be responsible for the two first aetiologies. By itself, hiatal hernia can cause symptoms without evidence of GERD[6]. The increased exposure of the oesophagus to gastric juice produces oesophagitis and stricture[5].

This disease must be treated medically at first. If no improvement is observed, a pathophysiological study of the GERD should be done.

Antireflux operations

The goal of the antireflux operation is to increase the efficacy of the LES and the cardia. Many different techniques have been developed, such as reconstruction of the angle of Hiss, angulation of the cardio–oesophageal junction with the ligament teres, and anterior, posterior or complete valvuloplasty[7–18].

Although each of these techniques gave good results in the hands of those who described them (or who performed them very frequently), a gradual consensus was developed recognizing the advantages of the techniques described by Belsey and Nissen[19,20].

Both of these procedures incorporate a portion of the distal oesophagus into the stomach to ensure that it will be affected by changes in intra-abdominal pressure through the intragastric pressure[21–23].

Nissen's technique initially consisted of the invagination of the oesophagus into a sleeve of the gastric wall obtained from the upper portion of the stomach and the fundus. The gastrosplenic vessels and the diaphragmatic hiatus were untouched. Numerous adaptations were subsequently applied to the original technique, such as closure of the hiatal orifice, more or less extensive mobilization of the fundus, modifications of the valve and variations of the length of the valve[24,25].

The technique presented here is from Nissen, involving the construction of a 2–3 cm long valve after mobilization of the great curvature of the stomach by section of several short gastric vessels. Reduction in the calibre of the hiatal orifice is accomplished with sutures through the two crura muscles.

Patient selection

Candidates for Nissen fundoplication suffer from documented pathological gastro-oesophageal reflux, with or without hiatal hernia[1,26,27]. All patients have had at least six months of medical/dietetic/postural treatment. They either have recurrence of symptoms when treatment is stopped, or have no relief of symptoms or oesophageal lesions despite treatment.

In these circumstances, an oesophageal function study is carried out. This includes endoscopy and biopsy, barium studies, oesophageal manometry and 24 hours pH monitoring (see Figure 9.1)[27–29].

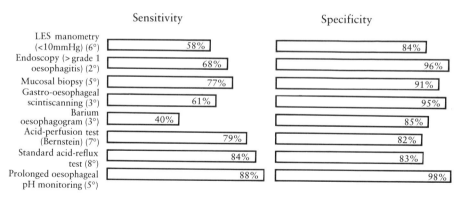

Figure 9.1: Example of an oesophageal study.

The indications to proceed with antireflux surgery are: documentation of a mechanically defective LES and increased exposure to gastric juice.

Some patients do have a large hiatal hernia: they complain mainly of dysphagia, chest pain and sometimes of heartburn[29]. The LES can be normal. A surgical repair will relieve the symptoms, but must be associated with an antireflux procedure because of the potential destruction of the competency of the cardio–oesophageal junction during the reduction of the hernia.

Criteria for acceptability for surgery are the same as for all abdominal surgery. A standard preanaesthetic investigation is done. The only surgical relative contraindications relate to previous gastric or hiatal surgery.

Laparoscopic Nissen fundoplication

Patient positioning

The operation is performed under general anaesthesia with endotracheal intubation; the patient is placed in the lithotomy position (*see* Figure 9.2).

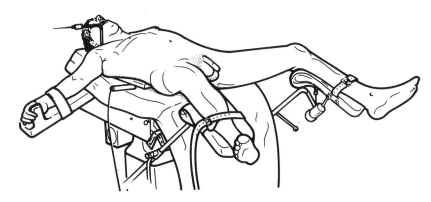

Figure 9.2: A patient in the Lloyd-Davis position.

The surgeon stands between the legs of his patient with the surgical assistant on his right and the scrub nurse or another assistant on his left (*see* Figure 9.3). The video–laparoscopy column is placed either on the right or the left of the surgeon.

Standard instruments are used (dissecting hook, curved scissors, atraumatic grasping forceps, Babcock forceps, clip applier, needle holder, dissecting forceps and palpators). A Penrose drain can be helpful. A monopolar cautery is attached to either the hook or the scissors. A 0° wide angle laparoscope is used.

Placement of trocars

Pneumoperitoneum is established in the normal fashion and with the usual precautions. A maximal intraperitoneal pressure of 15 mmHg is allowed.

The first trocar, 10 mm calibre, is placed in the supraumbilical midline at

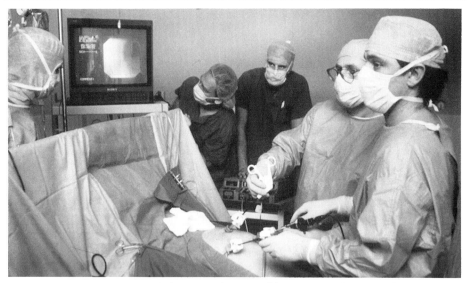

Figure 9.3: The surgeon stands between the legs of his patient, the surgical assistant on his right and the scrub nurse or another assistant on his left.

the junction of the upper two-thirds and lower third between the umbilicus and the xyphoid process. The laparoscope is introduced via this port. Visual inspection of the entire peritoneal cavity is carried out. Under direct vision, four other trocars are inserted: one 10 mm in the midline under the xyphoid process, and another 10 mm at the left upper quadrant at the mid-clavicular line, at a left paraumbilical position. Two 5 mm trocars are also used: one is placed under the right costal margin in the mid-clavicular line, and the other one laterally under the left costal margin on the anterior axillary line (*see* Figure 9.4).

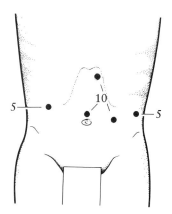

Figure 9.4: Trocar placement.

The use of 10 mm trocars allows maximal freedom to change the position of the laparoscope during the procedure, as well as the use of 10 mm instruments, such as the clip applier and certain needle holders and graspers.

Surgical procedure

This consists of:

- retraction of the left lobe of the liver using either an atraumatic forceps or a liver retractor introduced through the 5 mm right trocar (*see* Figure 9.5)

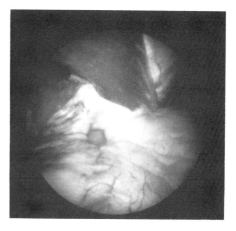

Figure 9.5: Retraction of the left lobe of the liver using either an atraumatic forceps or a liver retractor introduced through the 5 mm right trocar.

- division of the phreno–oesophageal membrane on the anterior aspect of the hiatal orifice. This incision is extended to the right to allow identification of the right crus. The dissection is carried out with the scissors introduced through the left paramedian port (*see* Figure 9.6)

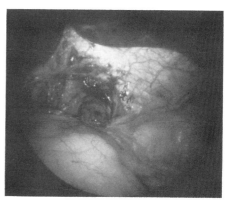

Figure 9.6: The dissection is carried out with the scissors introduced through the left paramedian port.

- liberation of the posterior aspect of the oesophagus by extending the dissection the length of the right diaphragmatic crus. The *pars flacida* of the lesser omentum is opened, preserving the hepatic branches of the vagus nerve. The posterior vagus nerve is identified (*see* Figure 9.7)

- incision of the gastrophrenic ligament and dissection of the left crus and left wall of the oesophagus (*see* Figure 9.8)

- intramediastinal dissection of the oesophagus to obtain an elongation of its intra-abdominal segment and a reduction of the hiatal hernia if it exists (*see* Figure 9.9)

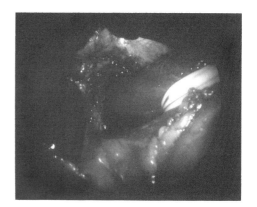

Figure 9.7: The *pars flacida* of the lesser omentum is opened, preserving the hepatic branches of the vagus nerve.

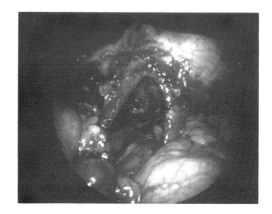

Figure 9.8 Incision of the gastrophrenic ligament and dissection of the left crus and left wall of the oesophagus.

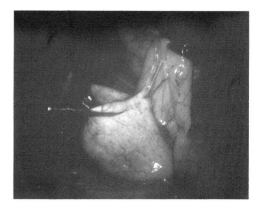

Figure 9.9: Intramediastinal dissection of the oesophagus obtains an elongation of the intra-abdominal segment and a reduction of the hiatal hernia.

- mobilization of the gastric pouch: this requires ligation and division of the gastrosplenic ligament and several short gastric vessels; two or three are clipped and divided, as required by the size of the fundus. This dissection starts on the stomach at the point where the vessels of the great curvature turn toward the spleen, away from the gastro-epiploic arcade (*see* Figure 9.10)

- retro-oesophageal dissection: the oesophagus is lifted by a forceps inserted

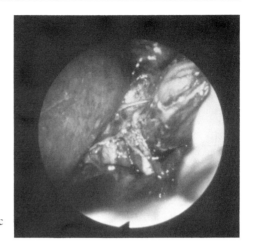

Figure 9.10: Mobilization of the gastric pouch.

through the left upper quadrant port. Careful dissection of the meso-oesophagus and the left crus reveals a cleavage plane between this crus and the posterior gastric wall. Confirmation of having opened the correct plane is obtained by visualizing the fatty tissue of the gastrosplenic ligament or the spleen itself, when looking behind the oesophagus. A rubber drain or Penrose drain can be used to lift up the oesophagus. This retro-oesophageal channel is enlarged to allow easy passage of the antireflux valve (*see* Figure 9.11)

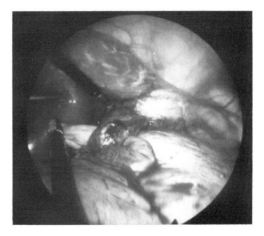

Figure 9.11: Retro-oesophageal dissection.

- repair of the hiatal orifice: two or three interrupted sutures, using non-absorbable material are placed on the diaphragmatic crura to close the orifice. A distance of approximately 1 cm must be maintained between the highest suture and the oesophagus (*see* Figure 9.11)

- passage and fixation of the antireflux valve: an atraumatic forceps is passed behind the oesophagus, from right to left. It is used to grab the gastric pouch to the left of the oesophagus and to pull it behind, forming the wrap (*see* Figure 9.12). At this point, a gastric tube (36–50 French) is passed down the cardia. It is used to calibrate the fundoplication.

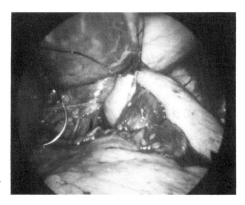

Figure 9.12: Passage and fixation of the antireflux valve.

Three to four interrupted stitches form and secure the sleeve. They are passed into the seromuscular layer of the anterior wall of the gastric pouch to the left of the oesophagus, through the seromuscular layer of the anterior oesophagus and, finally, to the right of the oesophagus, through the seromuscular layer of the stomach which had been passed behind the oesophagus. A 2–3 cm sleeve is constructed.

In some patients presenting with large sliding hiatal hernia, it is not always necessary to mobilize the fundus by cutting the short gastric vessels.

The large gastric tube is then replaced by a standard nasogastric tube. The peritoneum is lavaged with warm normal saline. No drains are placed. The cannulae are removed and the wounds are stapled closed.

Postoperative care

An intravenous line is left in place until the morning of the first postoperative day. The nasogastric tube is removed at the same time; the patient is then allowed to eat and drink.

On the second postoperative day, a barium study of the oesophagus, stomach and duodenum is carried out to verify the position and the function of the antireflux valve, as well as to confirm the absence of significant stenosis (*see* Figure 9.13). Afterwards the patient can be discharged. Dietary instructions are give to avoid the risk of impaction at the sleeve in the early postoperative period.

Conclusions

The operative technique presented is inspired from Nissen's original procedure[30]. The technique reproduces the same manoeuvres used in open procedure, with modifications for adaptation to laparoscopy.

The results obtained from a first series of 100 patients are similar, from

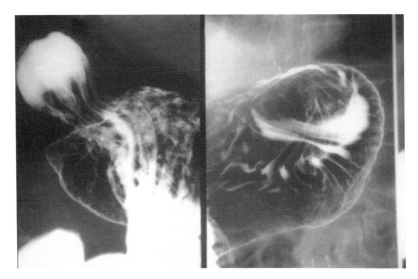

Figure 9.13: Barium study of the oesophagus, stomach and duodenum.

clinical (symptom reduction) as well as objective (manometric, endoscopic, radiological and photometric) standpoints, to those of the traditional procedure. The mortality rate is 0% and there have been no cases of splenic trauma. The postoperative period is eased by the laparoscopic approach, just as in cholecystectomy[31].

The initial long-term evaluations suggest a clear reduction in the classically described secondary effects of this operation, ie the gas bloat syndrome and dysphagia. Problems related to scar pain and to the abdominal wall, which handicap a certain number of patients after the open procedure, are eliminated.

The advantages of laparoscopic surgery are a significant reduction in hospital stay and an early return to professional and/or domestic life[30-33].

References

1   DeMeester TR and Stein HJ (1992) Surgical treatment of gastroesophageal reflux disease. In: Castell DO, ed. *The esophagus*. Little, Brown and Co., Boston.

2   Clarke J (1986) Hiatal hernia and reflux oesophagitis. In: Henessy TPJ and Cuschieri A, eds. *Surgery of the oesophagus*. Baillière Tindall, London.

3   Skinner BD (1985) Pathophysiology of gastroesophageal reflux. *Ann. Surg.* **206**:546–56.

4   DeMeester TR, Wernly JA and Bryant GH *et al.* (1979) Clinical and *in vitro* determinants of gastroesophageal competence: a study of the principles of antireflux surgery. *Am. J. Surg.* **137**:39–46.

5   Spechler SJ (1992) Complications of gastroesophageal reflux disease. In: Castell DO, ed. *The esophagus*. Little, Brown and Co., Boston.

6   Kerr RM (1992) Hiatal hernia and mucosal prolapse. In: Castell DO, ed. *The esophagus*. Little, Brown and Co., Boston.

7   Allison PR (1951) Reflux oesophagitis, sliding hiatus hernia and the anatomy of repair. *Surg. Gynecol. Obstet.* **92**:419–31.

8   Sweet RH (1952) Esophageal hiatus of the diaphragm. *Ann. Surg.* **135**:1–13.

9   Lortat-Jacob JL and Robert F (1953) Les malpositions cardio-tubérositaires. *Archives des Maladies de l'Appareil Digestif.* **42**:750–74.

10 Boerema I and Germs R (1955) Fixation of the lesser cure of the stomach to the anterior wall of the abdomen after reposition of the hernia through the oesophageal hiatus. *Archivum Chirurgicum Neerlandicum.* **7**:351–9.

11 Hill LD (1967) An effective operation for hiatal hernia: an eight year appraisal. *Ann. Surg.* **166**:681–92.

12 Toupet A (1963) Technique d'oesophago-gastroplastie avec phrenogastropexie appliquee dans la cure radicale des hernies hiatales et comme complement de l'operation de Heller dans les cardiospasmes. *Mem. Acad. Chir.* **89**:394.

13 Narbona-Arnau B, Molina E and Ancho-Fornos S *et al.* (1965) Hernia diaphragmatica hiatal. Pexia cardio-gastrica con el ligamento redondo. *Medicina de Espana.* **2**:25.

14 Thal AP, Hatafuku T and Kurtzman (1956) A new method for reconstruction of the esophagogastric junction. *Surg. Gynecol. Obstet.* **120**:1255.

15 Pearson FG, Cooper JD and Patterson GA *et al.* (1987) Gastroplasty and fundoplication for complex reflux problems. *Ann. Surg.* **206**:473–81

16 Watson A, Jenkinson LR and Ball CS *et al.* (1991) A more physiological alternative to total fundoplication for the surgical correction of resistant gastro-oesophageal reflux. *Br. J. Surg.* **78**:1088–94.

17 Woodward ER, Thomas HF and McAlhany JC (1971) Comparison of crural repair and Nissen fundoplication in the treatment of gastroesophageal reflux. *Ann. Surg.* **173**:782–92.

18 Thor KB and Silander T (1989) A long term randomized prospective trial of the Nissen procedure versus a modified Toupet technique. *Ann. Surg.* **210**:719–24.

19 DeMeester TR, Johnson LF and Kent AH (1974) Evaluation of current operations for the prevention of gastroesophageal reflux *Ann. Surg.* **180**:511–22.

20 Bombeck CT (1984) The choice of operations for gastroesophageal reflux. In: Watson A and Celestin LR, eds. *Disorders of the oesophagus*. Pitman Publishing, London.

21 Belsey R (1977) Surgical treatment of hiatus hernia and reflux esophagitis. *World J. Surg.* **1**:421–3.

22 Belsey R (1977) Mark IV repair of hiatal hernia by the transthoracic approach. *World J. Surg.* **1**:475–83.

23 Nissen R (1956) Eine einfache operation zur beeinflussung der refluxoesophagitis. *Schweiz. Med. Wochenschr.* **86**:590–2.

24 Rossetti M and Hell K (1977) Fundoplication for the treatment of gastro-esophageal reflux in hiatal hernia. *World J. Surg.* **1**:439–44.

25 DeMeester TR, Bonavina L and Albertucci M (1986) Nissen fundoplication for gastroesophageal reflux disease. Evaluation of primary repair in 100 consecutive patients. *Ann. Surg.* **204**:9–20.

26 Klinkenberg-Knol E and Castell DO (1992) Clinical spectrum and diagnosis of gastroesophageal reflux disease. In: Castell DO, ed. *The esophagus*. Little, Brown and Co., Boston.

27 DeMeester TR, Wang CI and Wernly JA *et al.* (1980) Technique, indications and clinical use of a 24-hour esophageal monitoring. *J. Thorac. Cardiovasc. Surg.* **79**:656–70.

28 Stein HJ, DeMeester TR and Naspetti R *et al.* (1991) Three dimensional imaging of the lower esophageal sphincter in gastroesophageal reflux disease. *Ann. Surg.* **214**:374–84.

29 Kaul BK, DeMeester TR and Oka M (1990) The cause of dysphagia in uncomplicated sliding hiatal hernia and its relief by hiatal herniorraphy. A Roentgenographic, manometric and clinical study. *Ann. Surg.* **211**:410–15.

30 Dallemagne B, Weerts JM and Jehaes C *et al.* (1991) Laparoscopic Nissen fundoplication. Preliminary report. *Surg. Laparosc. Surg.* **1**:138–43.

31 Dallemagne B, Weerts JM and Jehaes C *et al.* (1992) Cholecystectomie sous coelioscopie: analyse de 368 interventions. *Acta Gastr. Enterologica Belgica.* **55**:4–10.

32 Dallemagne B, Weerts JM and Jehaes C *et al.* (1993) Case report: subtotal esophagectomy by thoracoscopy and laparoscopy. *Minimally Invasive Therapy* (In press).

33 Dallemagne B, Weerts JM and Jehaes C *et al.* (1990) Douleurs abdominales: coelioscopie et chirurgie per-coelioscopique. *Rev. Med. Liège.* **XLV**:152–6.

10

Endoscopic Oesophagectomy

BERNARD DALLEMAGNE AND JOSEPH M. WEERTS

Anatomic review

The oesophagus is a muscular tube extending from the pharynx to the stomach, and varying in length between 25 and 30 cm. For endoscopy, the length is measured from the dental arcade. Using this reference, its length is 40 cm in men and between 35 and 37 cm in women (*see* Figure 10.1). At the cervical level, the oesophagus lies between the trachea in front and the prevertebral fascia behind. The recurrent laryngeal nerves are found on either side in the groove separating the trachea from the oesophagus.

The same anterior and posterior relations hold true in the thorax, down to the level of the tracheal bifurcation, at the fifth thoracic vertebra. Below this, the oesophagus is related anteriorly to the left main bronchus, the pericardium and the left atrium.

Below the carina, various structures are found posteriorly between the oesophagus and the vertebral bodies: the azygos vein, the thoracic duct and the descending aorta. The azygos vein runs along the right side of the vertebral column, then crosses the oesophagus at the level of the right pulmonary hilum to drain into the superior vena cava. The thoracic duct is found behind the oesophagus and crosses its left border obliquely above the aortic arch. The descending thoracic aorta progressively crosses behind the oesophagus initially on the left, and finishes on the right posterolateral aspect above the diaphragm.

The vagus nerves descend with the oesophagus below the carina and remain adherent through the hiatal passage, where the oesophagus is invested by the gastrophrenic ligament.

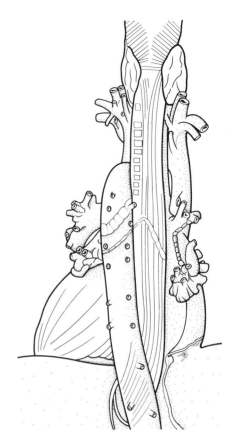

Figure 10.1: Anatomical relationship of the oesophagus in the thorax. (Reprinted with permission from Sobotta J and Becher H, eds (1973) *Atlas der Anatomie des Menschen*. Urban and Schwartzenberg, Berlin.)

Techniques of oesophagectomy

One treatment for oesophageal cancer is oesophagectomy. This is only performed for resectable tumours; surgical palliative techniques will not be discussed in this chapter.

In order to establish resectability, a detailed preoperative investigation is necessary to exclude local and/or distant extension. Local spread is detected by endoluminal techniques (endoscopy with biopsies), and by medical imaging including chest X-ray, thoracomediastinal computed tomography (CT) scan and echo endoscopy. Distant spread is diagnosed using abdominal ultrasound, abdominal CT scan and also endoluminal ultrasonography with examination of the coeliac trunk for adenopathy. More precise staging is possible with laparoscopy and thoracoscopy prior to surgical resection.

Once resectability has been established, one of two traditional surgical approaches may be used for oesophagectomy: thoracotomy or transhiatal dissection.

Left thoracotomy can be performed with intrathoracic anastomosis (the Sweet technique[1]) or a right-sided approach. Here intrathoracic[2] or cervical anastomosis is carried out. The substitution tube is brought up either through the mediastinum or retrosternally[3–10].

Transhiatal dissection of the oesophagus theoretically allows reduction in perioperative pulmonary damage and postoperative pain[4,5]. The technique was therefore primarily indicated for patients with major compromise pulmonary function, and with tumour limited to the oesophageal wall or easily accessible lesions (lower third of the oesophagus).

Until recently, these two approaches were the only means of accomplishing oesophageal resection. In 1989, however, Buess[6,7] introduced the technique of transcervical endoscopic dissection: a modified rigid endoscope is introduced into the mediastinum via a left cervical approach. This allows progressive dissection of the entire length of the oesophagus while avoiding the trauma of thoracotomy and the danger of blind transhiatal dissection.

The advantage of open techniques is that they allow wide mediastinectomy, with removal of not only the oesophagus but also the entire perioesophageal lymphatic system. This has importance for the long-term results of the surgery[8,9].

The advent of surgical laparoscopy of the digestive tract inspired surgeons to use this instrument in the thorax to dissect out the oesophagus. This technique combines the advantages of thoracotomy (completeness of excision and lymphatic dissection) with those of closed thorax techniques (preservation of ventilatory mechanics).

The thoracoscopic oesophagectomy is combined with an abdominal approach to prepare a substitutive organ; the abdominal phase can be carried out in the traditional way, with laparotomy or laparoscopy.

The anastomosis between the 'neo-oesophagus' and the oesophageal stump is performed through a left cervicotomy.

The intrathoracic anastomosis can be carried out using mechanical staplers; although these techniques have not yet been clinically applied and will not be described here.

Operative technique

Subtotal oesophagectomy is carried out in two phases: thoracic via thoracoscopy and abdominocervical. Patients are intubated with a double lumen endotracheal tube to allow one-lung ventilation.

Thoracoscopy

POSITIONING–SURGICAL APPROACH
The patient is positioned as for a right thoracotomy and left lung ventilation is initiated. The operating surgeon stands to the patient's right, with an assistant on either side. The video monitor is placed facing the surgeon.

A 10 mm thoracic trocar is placed in the right sixth intercostal space at the midaxillary line. A 0° wide angled telescope is introduced via this port and an initial evaluation of the lung and pleural cavity is carried out.

Four more thoracic trocars and cannulae are inserted under direct vision: their position depends somewhat on each patient's anatomy. Two trocars,

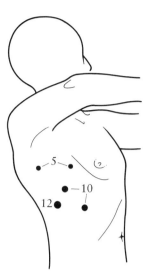

Figure 10.2: Sites of trocar insertion in the chest.

5 mm and 10 mm respectively, are placed in the anterior axillary line and two others (5 mm and 12 mm) on the posterior axillary line (Figure 10.2). The 10 mm trocars allow the telescope to be moved and a clip applier to be used. The 12 mm trocar is used to dissect and use the mechanical stapler. No insufflation is necessary. The surgeon uses atraumatic grasping forceps and dissecting scissors attached to electrocautery via the posterior ports. The telescopic videocamera is held by an assistant, either on the right or left, depending on the phase of the dissection. The assistant on the surgeon's right also controls a suction cannula introduced via the inferior port in the anterior axillary line. The assistant on the left holds a lung retractor introduced through the superior port on the same line.

OESOPHAGEAL DISSECTION

Division of the triangular ligament down to the inferior pulmonary vein allows retraction of the right lung (*see* Figure 10.3) At this stage, resectability can once again be assessed, especially in terms of local extension into mediastinal structures.

The mediastinal pleura is opened: posteriorly along the azygos vein and, above its arch, along the rightmost aspect of the spine; then anteriorly, along the pericardium, the inferior pulmonary vein, the right main bronchus and the trachea. The pleural incisions meet at the apex of the pleural cavity and at the hiatal aperture.

The dissection of the oesophagus starts at the diaphragmatic hiatus. If the abdominal phase is to be performed using laparoscopy, the hiatus should not be opened. The dissection is carried out in the traditional way:

- posteriorly: the thoracic duct is clipped and divided. The dissection is continued following the periaortic periadventitium as far as the left pleura (*see* Figure 10.4). The mediastinectomy is extended to the

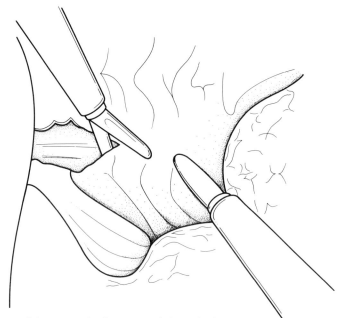

Figure 10.3: Section of the triangular ligament of the right lung.

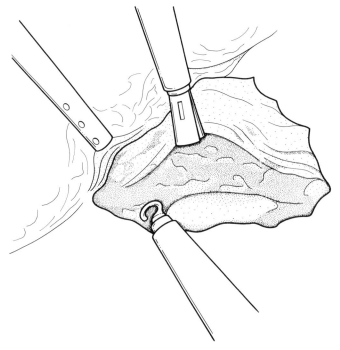

Figure 10.4: Incision of the posterior pleura on the anterior border of the aorta.

level of the aortic arch; at this level, the arch of the azygos vein is divided using the EndoGIA (US Surgical Corporation, Connecticut) introduced through the 12 mm port (*see* Figure 10.5). Further dissection proceeds by clipping and coagulating small oesophagobronchial branches.

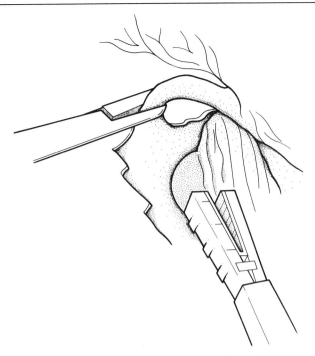

Figure 10.5: Transection of the azygos arch using a mechanical stapler (EndoGIA, US Surgical Corporation, Connecticut).

- anteriorly: the dissection follows the pericardium as far as the left pleura. It proceeds upward, behind the inferior pulmonary vein and the right main bronchus; here the right bronchial artery, originating from the right intercostal artery and crossing the oesophagus, must be clipped. The posterior bronchial plane is followed as far as the left main bronchus. The intertracheaobronchial nodes are removed, followed by division of the right vagus nerve. The dissection then proceeds along the posterior aspect of the trachea. This anteroposterior dissection can be facilitated by isolating the oesophagus with a sling. This renders the dissection of the left aspect easier.

- on the left: the dissection extends upwards following the plane of the pleura to the inferior aspect of the aortic arch.

The left recurrent laryngeal nerve must be identified before dividing the left vagus. Above the aortic arch, the pleural plane is once again followed.

The mediastinectomy concludes the thoracic phase. Warm saline lavage and verification of haemostasis is followed by placement of a chest tube via the orifice of the 12 mm trocar. Its position is confirmed by thoracoscopy and the right lung is re-expanded. The cutaneous orifices are stapled shut.

Abdominocervical phase

POSITIONING–SURGICAL APPROACH
The patient is placed supine. The legs are spread (in laparoscopy) or left

together on the table (in laparotomy). The left cervical area is prepared and draped.

LAPAROTOMY

A standard laparotomy incision is made. The peritoneal cavity is explored, looking for cardiac, gastric, coeliac and hepatic adenopathy. This exploration allows a decision to be made as to whether or not the stomach can be used as a substitution organ. This is especially important for adenocarcinomas of the lower third of the oesophagus. The abdominal exploration can be carried out prior to the thoracic phase, especially using laparoscopy.

The abdominal phase is then carried out conventionally, with:

- liberation of the greater curvature of the stomach

- liberation of the abdominal oesophagus and the cardia

- removal of coeliac lymph nodes

- gastroplasty.

At the beginning of the gastroplasty, a second surgical team begins the cervical phase, with:

- oblique incision along the anterior border of the sternocleidomastoid muscle, or skin crease just above the clavicle

- posterior retraction of the left jugulocarotid bundle

- dissection of the oesophagus by its left aspect and isolation by a rubber band securing a nasogastric tube to the distal end of the oesophagus.

The operative specimen is removed through the abdomen via the diaphragmatic hiatus. This brings the nasogastric tube into the abdomen; it is later used to guide the gastroplasty through the mediastinum. After bringing the gastroplasty into the neck, a cervical anastomosis is performed. The cervical incision is then closed.

A pylorotomy or plasity is carried out; Kocher's manoeuvre is used to minimize tension on the gastroplasty, and the abdominal incision is closed.

With laparotomy, the conventional variations can be used: right or left with colonic interposition, total gastric ascension and retrosternal trajectory[10].

LAPAROSCOPY

The patient is placed in the lithotomy position, with the legs held in stirrups or on a split table. The surgeon is positioned between the patient's legs with an assistant at either side. The video system is placed to the patient's right.

Preparing and draping for a left cervicotomy are also performed at this point. A pneumoperitoneum in induced by insufflation of carbon dioxide via a Verres needle introduced into the left upper quadrant. The high-flow electronic insufflator is programmed to a maximal pressure of 15 mmHg. A 10 mm trocar is introduced via the umbilicus. The 0° wide angle laparoscope is inserted and an initial evaluation of the peritoneal cavity is carried out (stomach, liver, peritoneal surface) looking for metastatic lesions.

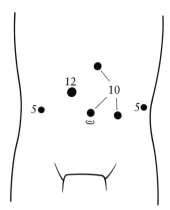

Figure 10.6: Sites of trocars insertion on the abdomen (laparoscopic stage).

Four other trocars and cannulae are inserted, arranged for laparoscopic surgery of the stomach and hiatal orifice: a 5 mm port is placed at the left costal margin along the anterior axillary line. A second 5 mm port is inserted at the right costal margin at the mid-clavicular line. Two other 10 mm ports are inserted, one in the upper third of the midline between the xiphoid process and the umbilicus, and the second at the left mid-clavicular line, midway between the costal margin and the umbilicus.

A 12 mm trocar will be inserted into the right paraxyphoid area when the gastric tube is being performed (*see* Figure 10.6).

The stages of the abdominal phase are identical to those during laparotomy.

Gastrolysis. The gastrocolic ligament is opened, allowing entry into the omental bursa. It is then divided parallel to the greater curvature of the stomach, respecting the gastroepiploic arcade (*see* Figure 10.7). This dissection is carried out with the coagulating hook and surgical clips. It is extended towards the right gastroepiploic pedicle. Towards the left, the left gastroepiploic vessels are clipped and divided. The gastrolysis is continued

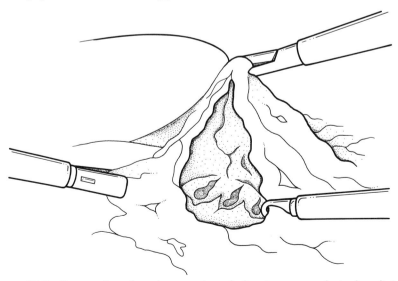

Figure 10.7: Preparation for the gastric tubulization: gastrolysis by dividing the gastrohepatic and gastrocolic ligaments, preserving the right gastric artery and the right gastric epiploic vascular arcade along the greater curvature of the stomach.

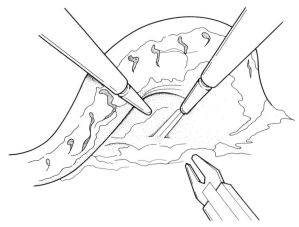

Figure 10.8: Division of the left gastric vessels by lifting up the stomach.

along the greater curvature by division of the gastrosplenic ligament after clipping and cutting the short vessels.

The hiatus is not opened at this stage of the operation: this would lead to loss of the pneumoperitoneum into the pleural cavity.

Coeliac dissection. The stomach is lifted, putting tension on the left gastric vessels at the superior margin of the pancreas. The retroperitoneum is incised at this point, and the gastric artery and vein are clipped and divided (*see* Figure 10.8). The dissection is continued upward to the diaphragmatic crura. At the level of the lesser curvature, the vascular arcade is sectioned using a vascular stapler at the level of the crow's foot. This is where the gastroplasty will begin.

Gastroplasty. The stomach is tubed using a mechanical stapler introduced through the right paramedian 12 mm port.

Use of successive cartridge allows creation of the gastric tube starting from the foot of the lesser curve and ending at the fundus. The path is parallel to the greater curvature, with a width of approximately 3 cm (*see* Figures 10.9 and 10.10).

Hiatal opening. When the gastric tube is finished, attention is turned to the diaphragmatic orifice. The classic cervical phase is started at this point. The phreno–oesophageal membrane is incised on the anterior wall of the oesophagus. The dissection is continued toward the right crus to join that which was done in the retrogastric phase. The left crus is also dissected allowing complete mobilization of the oesophagus.

The patient's haemodynamic and ventilatory status must be evaluated carefully when the hiatus is opened, with consequent loss of peritoneal gas into the mediastinum and right pleural cavity.

Specimen extraction. The gastroplasty is secured to the proximal stomach. The specimen, including the oesophagus and the proximal stomach, is removed via the cervicotomy. The gastroplasty follows into the mediastinum (*see* Figure 10.11). Laparoscopy is used to ensure correct positioning.

Cervical suture. After verifying easy passage of a nasogastric tube, the cervical route is used to perform a conventional oesophagogastric suture.

Warm saline lavage and verification of haemostasis are carried out in the abdominal cavity. The pneumoperitoneum is released, the cannulae are withdrawn and the cutaneous puncture sites are closed.

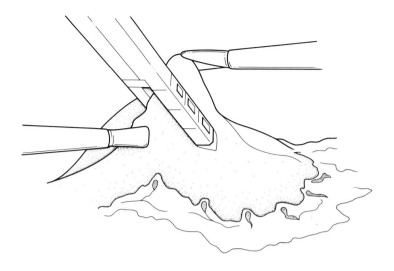

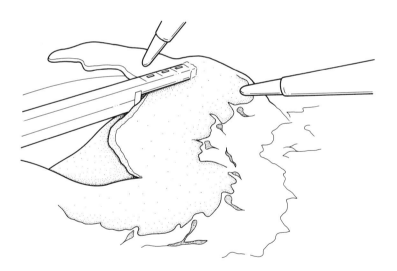

Figure 10.9 and 10.10: Tubulization of the stomach by using mechanical stapler applied parallel to the greater gastric curvature, at a distance of approximately 2.5 cm.

Postoperative care

The patient is nursed in the intensive care unit. Mechanical ventilation is continued for 12–24 hours. Daily chest X-rays are performed to follow the possible appearance of pulmonary complications. Chest physiotherapy is started immediately, with full patient co-operation as soon as he is extubated.

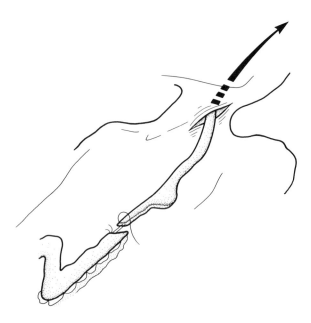

Figure 10.11: Extraction of the specimen (proximal part of the stomach and the oesophagus) through the left cervical incision.

This is facilitated if the surgery has been carried out with 'scopy'; by the near absence of thoracic (and abdominal) pain. Non-opiate analgesia is used for the first three or four postoperative days.

On the fourth postoperative day, a contrast study of the oesophagus, stomach and duodenum is carried out using hydro-soluble material. If the result is positive, the patient is allowed to drink and is discharged to the regular ward.

Conclusions

Two new techniques – transcervical dissection and thoracoscopy – have recently been added to the traditional techniques of oesophagectomy (trans-hiatal approach and thoracotomy).

The advantages of the newer techniques lie in the spectacular reduction in pulmonary trauma. The precision and extent of the dissection with thoracoscopy are equal to those of thoracotomy, because the same steps are carried out. The newer techniques can be used with 'classic' laparotomy; on the other hand thoracoscopy can be combined with a laparoscopic abdominal phase, with its universally recognized advantages[11].

The reduced surgical trauma of the endoscopic technique may have an impact on long-term survival. Evaluation of this hypothesis requires the careful follow-up of an organized series of patients.

References

1   Sweet RH, Soutar L and Tejala Valenzuela C (1954) Muscle wall tumors of the esophagus. *J. Thorac. Surg.* **27**:13–35.

2   Lewis I (1946) The surgical treatment of carcinoma of the oesophagus with special reference to a new operation for the growths of the middle third. *Br. J. Surg.* **34**:18–25.

3   Akiyama H, Tsurumaru M, Kawamura T and Ono Y (1981) Principles of surgical treatment for carcinoma of the esophagus. Analysis of lymph node involvement. *Ann. Surg.* **194**:438–43.

4   Orringer MB and Sloan H (1978) Esophagectomy without thoracotomy. *Thorac. Cardiovasc. Surg.* **76**:643–54.

5   Baker JW and Schechter GL (1986) Management of esophageal cancer by blunt resection without thoracotomy and reconstruction with stomach. *Ann. Surg.* **203**:491–9.

6   Kipfmuller K, Naruhn M, Melzer A, Kessler S and Buess G (1989) Endoscopic microsurgical dissection of the esophagus: results in animal model. *Surg. Endosc.* **3**:63–9.

7   Buess GF, Becker HD, Naruhn MB *et al.* (1991) Endoscopic esophagectomy without thoracotomy. *Problems in Gen. Surg.* **8**:478–86.

8   Skinner DB, Little AG and Ferguson MK *et al.* (1986) Selection of operation for esophageal cancer based on staging. *Ann. Surg.* **204**:391–401.

9   Tam PC, Siu KF, Cheung HC, Ma L and Wong J (1987) Local recurrences after subtotal esophagectomy for squamous cell carcinoma. *Ann. Surg.* **205**:189–94.

10 DeMeester TR and Stein HJ (1992) Surgical therapy for cancer of the esophagus and cardia. In: Castell DO ed. *The esophagus*. Little, Brown and Co., Boston.

11 Dallemagne B, Weerts JM and Jehaes C *et al.* (1992) Case report: subtotal oesophagectomy by thoracoscopy and laparoscopy. *Min. Inv. Ther.* **1**:183–5.

11

Thoracoscopic Sympathectomy

JOHN A. RENNIE

Hyperhidrosis is a pathological condition affecting young people. The sweating is in excess of that required for thermoregulation and is usually manifest in the hands, axillae and feet. Occasionally, the face and trunk are also involved. The hands alone are involved in 20%, the hands and axillae in 43% and the axillae alone in 37% of cases[1].

Hyperhidrosis may be socially disabling. Typists and VDU workers, hairdressers, shop assistants, musicians and receptionists all find the cold clammy hand of the hyperhidrotic a source of great embarrassment, and young patients desperately seek treatment, usually from dermatologists.

Hyperhidrosis is usually primary, but may be secondary to thyrotoxicosis and phaechromocytoma, with an overall incidence of 0.6–1.0%[2]. Medical treatments with probanthine, biofeedback techniques[3] and iontopheresis[4] are characterized by complications, short-lived effects and disappointed patients.

Local excision of sweat glands leaves a badly scarred axilla and stiffness of the shoulder joint[5]. Sympathectomy remains the gold standard against which all treatments must be measured. Various operative approaches have been advocated, all of which must be judged against the simplest and least complicated – the endoscopic method.

The supraclavicular[6], posterior[7] and transaxillary[8] methods, whilst still practised, have been superseded by the endoscopic method[9]. This is simple to learn, efficacious and allows the procedure to be performed in a day unit.

Technique

All patients should have a preoperative chest X-ray to exclude any pulmonary disease which may hinder the establishment of a pneumothorax.

The procedure is performed under general anaesthetic, ideally with a double lumen tube. An endotracheal tube is sufficient if skilled anaesthesia is not available[10]. The patient is placed in a supine position with both arms abducted to 60°.

Once the appropriate lung has been deflated, an artificial pneumothorax is established using a Verres needle inserted through the fourth intercostal space. Two litres of carbon dioxide are slowly insufflated into the pleural space. Rapid introduction of gas at this stage may produce a profound brachycardia as the mediastinum is shifted away from the needle. Through the same 0.5 cm incision, a 5 mm laparoscope is then inserted through a cannula and advanced across the pleural cavity under direct vision, until the ribs are identified (*see* Figures 11.1–11.3). The ribs are then followed medially until the sympathetic ganglia and chain are seen over the necks of the ribs. The highest rib seen on either side is the second. Care must be taken in the right chest (*see* Figure 11.3). The azygos vein may lie close to the sympathetic ganglia and may be of considerable diameter. Careful diathermy incision of the pleura along the lateral border of the azygos vein may be necessary to expose the sympathetic chain fully. The operating table may be rotated to the 'anti-Trendelenberg' (head up) position to decompress the veins, and to expose the fourth and fifth ribs.

During the visualization of the ganglia, pleural adhesions may need to be divided. Carbon dioxide should slowly be introduced via the cannula at no greater pressure than 20 mmHg.

A separate stab incision in the anterior axillary line through the fifth intercostal space allows the introduction of a diathermy probe via an insulated cannula. By pushing with the probe, the ganglia – with their soft consistency and glistening surface – can be positively identified. Each ganglion is destroyed with a low unipolar diathermy current until the bare rib is seen in the base of the cavity. The fifth ganglion may be ablated if axillary hyperhidrosis is present. Finally, the interconnecting rami between the ganglia can be gently diathermied, care being taken not to diathermy above the second rib. Haemostasis at this stage must be secured.

The diathermy probe and cannula are then removed and the laparoscope held ready while the lung is reinflated. Full inflation of the lung is checked by reinserting the laparoscope and observing the size of pneumothorax. If the lung has reinflated, the laparoscope and cannula are removed and the wound sealed with a stitch or steristrip. A chest X-ray should be performed in the recovery area to check for residual pneumothorax. A small pneumothorax is acceptable and is usually reabsorbed within 24 hours. Chest drains are not used routinely.

The patient is returned to the ward and usually discharged the following day.

Single or bilateral?

With a careful technique, ensuring that the pneumothorax has been adequately reduced, there is no good reason why the procedure may not be performed bilaterally at one operation. Strict attention to haemostasis must be observed, but time for both operations is rarely more than 20 minutes.

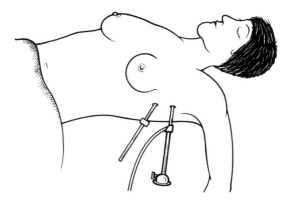

Figure 11.1: Through the same 0.5 cm incision, a 5 mm laparoscope is inserted through a cannula and advanced across the pleural cavity under direct vision, until the ribs are identified.

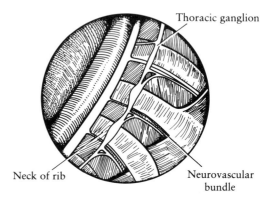

Thoracic ganglion

Neck of rib

Neurovascular bundle

Figure 11.2: View of left thoracic sympathectomy.

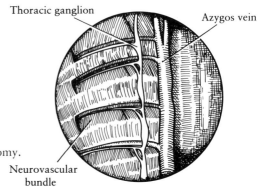

Thoracic ganglion

Azygos vein

Neurovascular bundle

Figure 11.3: View of right thoracic sympathectomy.

Intrapleural drainage

This is not usually required. The chest X-ray at the end of the procedure, usually performed in the recovery area, may show a small residual apical pneumothorax. If the patient's vital signs are satisfactory, a small pneumothorax can be ignored as resorption of this gas takes place over the following 24 hours.

If a significant pneumothorax is noted, or damage to the lung is suspected, a fine pleural drain can be inserted through one of the incisions in the anterior axillary line, and thence connected to an underwater seal. This may usually be removed at 24 hours if the lung has reinflated on a subsequent chest X-ray.

The frequency with which chest drains are required compares favourably with the open method. Greenhalgh[11] reported the need for a chest drain in 26% of cases by the open method; Byrne[12] reported one in 85 patients, and we needed three chest drains in a series of 77 patients[13].

Horner's syndrome

This was one of the most distressing complications of the open method of sympathectomy. Damage to the stellate ganglion, either by ablation or dissection, renders the patient permanently deformed.

Laparoscopic sympathectomy has virtually abolished this complication, because the highest rib that can be directly viewed intrapleurally via the laparoscope is the second rib. Diathermy of the ganglion over the neck of the highest and most easily viewed rib is safe, and Horner's should not occur.

In my personal series of 77 sympathectomies to date, I have recorded three cases of transient Horner's syndrome. Two were early in the series, probably due to using too high a diathermy current for the ablation. Heat, conducted along the nerves, will cause a neuropraxia of the stellate ganglion. The patient can be reassured about its transient nature, and full recovery can be confidently expected.

Again, the incidence of Horner's syndrome by the endoscopic method compares favourably with the open method. Greenhalgh[11] reported a 14% incidence and Adar[2] a 57% incidence of Horner's syndrome by the open method. Byrne[12] reported three in a series of 85 patients and we had three cases of transient Horner's syndrome in a series of 77 by the laparoscopic method[13].

Indications for thoracic sympathectomy

There is one absolute indication for this procedure – disabling hyperhidrosis. Experience over 15 years in a number of centres suggests that the results are highly predictable and apparently permanent.

Relative indications remain: Raynaud's disease, digital ischaemia and causalgia. The results in Raynaud's disease are temporary, for within six to 12 months the vasospasm returns, presumably mediated by some as yet unrecognized non-adrenergic, non-cholinergic stimulatory nerve fibres.

Compensatory hyperhidrosis

All patients undergoing a sympathectomy procedure should be warned that compensatory hyperhidrosis occurs in approximately 50% of patients[1,15]. Its mechanism is unknown and appears to be a problem for those who suffer from extreme hyperhidrosis of hands, axillae and feet.

Compensatory hyperhidrosis manifests itself as excessive sweating over parts of the body where sweating was not noticeable prior to thoracic sympathectomy. The usual sites are the trunk and thighs but there has been at least one case of the head being affected.

Postal questionnaires have been conducted and, whilst compensatory hyperhidrosis is a recognized complication in 50% of patients, few felt it worthy of complaint[13]. Most patients accepted the problem and were glad to have dry hands and axillae.

Comparison of the open and endoscopic techniques reveals a similar incidence of this complication.

The cause of compensatory sweating remains contentious. Monro[16] believed a latent reflex was activated by sympathectomy and Byrne[12] showed that 60% of his patients had a precipitating cause. Others believe it to be a response associated with heat regulation. Guttman[17] was the first to describe 'perilesionary' hyperhidrosis, and Shelley[14] calculated that 40% of sweat gland formation is lost with bilateral thoracic sympathectomy. In our series, only the severest hyperhidrotics were affected[13]. The sequence of events after bilateral thoracic sympathectomy is of relevance. Compensatory sweating usually develops within days of the sympathectomy and often in response to a stimulus, such as exertion, stress or food. However, gustatory sweating may not occur for several months. This can be explained by sprouting of regenerating sympathetic nerves. This process may produce aberrant innervation between sympathetic nerves and the cholinergic supply, involving either the salivary glands and/or the vagus.

Gustatory sweating

This may occur in association with compensatory sweating. In our postal survey, 48% of patients noted some symptoms (although no actual sweating) related to a variety of foods, especially cheese and spicy foods.

Postoperative pain

The pain experienced after the operation varies considerably. Five patients in our postal survey complained of pain which commenced between 24 and 48 hours postoperatively and which was predominantly in the back. The delay in onset of the pain and the distribution is suggestive of a perichondritis, secondary to the diathermy ablation of the ganglion over the neck of the rib.

Pain was controlled with non-steroidal anti-inflammatory drugs and had resolved completely in all cases within 20 days.

A notable feature of the transaxillary approach is the postoperative pain, particularly if a portion of the rib is resected for access[8]. In our questionnaire, however, the lack of any pain associated with the procedure was noted by the majority. 70% returned to work within a week and began playing their usual sports within two weeks.

Subjective assessment

Questionnaires were sent to 50 patients after a mean follow-up of 26 months (3–55 months). The mean age was 29.3 years, and the range was 16–59 years.

Complications such as compensatory sweating and gustatory sweating were noted, but they were considered to be less distressing than the original sweating by the majority, and only one patient has warranted further investigation.

Hyperhidrosis of the hands can be treated confidently by this method and an almost 100% success rate can be predicted. The axilla can be improved by 70–80% by this method, although it does demand ablation of the fifth ganglion which may be difficult to visualize.

Lower limb hyperhidrosis can now be treated by phenol lumbar sympathetic block.

Conclusion

An endoscopic approach to ablation of the thoracic sympathetic ganglion for the treatment of upper limb hyperhidrosis is now well tried and effective. Complications are minimal and the effect is permanent, but all patients should be warned of the possibility of developing compensatory hyperhidrosis.

References

1   Kux M (1978) Thoracic endoscopic sympathectomy in palmar and axillary hyperhidrosis. *Arch. Surg.* **113**:264–6.

2   Adar R, Kurchin A, Zweig A and Mozes M (1977) Palmar hyperhidrosis and its surgical treatment. *Ann. Surg.* **186**:34–41.

3   Duller P and Doyle Gentry W (1980) Use of biofeedback in treating chronic hyperhidrosis: a preliminary report. *Br. J. Dermatol.* **103**:143.

4   Midtgaard K (1986) A new device for the treatment of hyperhidrosis by iontopheresis. *Br. J. Dermatol.* **114**:485–8.

5   Breach NM (1979) Axillary hyperhidrosis: surgical cure with aesthetic scars. *Ann. R. Coll. Surg. Engl.* **61**:295–7.

6   Telford ED (1935) The technique of sympathectomy. *Br. J. Surg.* **23**:448–50.

7   Adson AW and Brown GE (1932) Extreme hyperhidrosis of the hands and feet treated by sympathetic ganglionectomy. *Mayo Clin. Proc.* **7**:394.

8   Atkins MJB (1949) Peraxillary approach to the stellate and upper thoracic sympathetic ganglion. *Lancet.* ii:1152

9   Malone PS, Cameron AEP and Rennie JA (1986) Endoscopic thoracic sympathectomy in the treatment of upper limb hyperhidrosis. *Annals R.C.S.* **68**:93–4.

10   Weale FE (1980) Upper thoracic sympathectomy by transthoracic electrocoagulation. *Br. J. Surg.* **67**:71–2.

11   Greenhalgh RM, Rosengarten DS and Martin P (1971) Role of sympathectomy for hyperhidrosis. *Br. Med. J.* **1**:332–4.

12   Byrne J, Walsh TN and Hederman WP (1990) Endoscopic transthoracic electrocautery of the sympathetic chain for palmar and axillary hyperhidrosis. *Br. J. Surg.* **77**:1046–9.

13   Edmondson RA, Bannerjee AK and Rennie JA (1992) Endoscopic transthoracic sympathectomy in the treatment of hyperhidrosis. *Ann. Surg.* **215**:289–93.

14   Shelley WB and Florence R (1960) Compensatory hyperhidrosis after sympathectomy. *N. Engl. J. Med.* **263**:1056–8.

15   Bogokowsky M, Slutzki S, Bacami L, Abrahamson R and Negri M (1983) The surgical treatment of primary hyperhidrosis. *Arch. Surg.* **118**:1065–7.

16   Monro PAG (1959) *Sympathectomy: an anatomical and physiological study with clinical applications.* Oxford University Press, Oxford.

17   Guttman L (1940) Distribution of disturbances of sweat secretion after extirpation of certain sympathetic cervical ganglia in man. *J. Anat.* **72**:537–49.

12

Endoscopic Colonic Surgery

PATRICK F. LEAHY

The widespread popularization of endoscopic surgery since 1989 has prompted many surgeons to explore the potential advantages of endoscopic bowel surgery. Central to their enthusiasm is the great improvement in technological assistance in the form of both video optics and instrumentation. There is now a widespread belief that investment in advanced technology video-assisted surgery will ultimately help to reduce the overall burden of health care in the United States, Europe and Asia.

Patient selection

In selecting patients for endoscopic bowel surgery, the surgeon must adhere to the already established criteria for colonic resection for benign and malignant disease. An additional stipulation for the aspiring endoscopic surgeon is to confine his attention to patients with benign disease until he has acquired the necessary skill to effect a superior cancer operation. Once the expertise to perform endoscopic bowel surgery has been acquired, the surgeon could comply with the established guidelines for selection of patients with carcinoma and phlegmaneous diverticular disease.

Preoperative preparation

All patients who have endoscopic bowel surgery should be informed of the inherent risks and advantages of such a procedure. It is also mandatory to enlighten patients about situations where it may be deemed necessary to perform a laparotomy incision. The patient is placed on a low-fibre diet for one week prior to surgery. Three days prior to surgery he is advised to increase his oral liquid intake and reduce solid intake; 48 hours before surgery he will be maintained on a normal liquid diet with elemental diet supplements. One day prior to surgery he is commenced on the standard Go Lytely bowel preparation.

Patient positioning

The patient is placed in a supine position on the operating table. General anaesthesia is administered and endotracheal intubation is effected. A Foley catheter is inserted and a nasogastric tube is inserted into the patient's stomach. The patient is placed on Lloyd Davis leg stirrups and these are placed in a slightly abducted position. The abdomen and perineum are prepared and appropriate draping for low anterior resection is effected. The patient is placed in a 30° Trendelenberg position.

Instrumentation

In this operation a preference may be shown for the use of laser. The most effective laser for this form of advanced surgical technique is an Nd:YAG or Ho:YAG laser, which should be placed behind the operating surgeon. In some cases, especially in low anterior resections and operations involving dissection in the presacral plexus of veins, an argon beam coagulator is useful (Beacon, Valley Lab., Bircher).

It is imperative that intestinal clamps or Babcocks are available for grasping the bowel. The available intestinal clamps are 5 mm clamps (Glassman, Dorcey). In addition to the laser, accurate and precise dissection can be achieved using monopolar electrocautery in combination with sharp disposable dissecting scissors, eg endoshears (US Surgical Corporation, Connecticut). A second light source is used in combination with a 10 mm 30° side-viewing telescope to transilluminate the mesenteric arcade. The light source should be a halogen or zenon light source with a power wattage of at least 150–300 W. A modified Babcock device grasps and removes the trocar from the PCEEA (US Surgical Corporation) and also grasps the anvil of the stapling device.

Positioning of trocars

A four puncture technique is used in the majority of cases of low anterior resection (*see* Figure 12.1). A 10 mm port is placed in the right upper quadrant, three finger breadths above the umbilicus. A 12 mm port is placed in the right lower quadrant to facilitate entry of the EndoGIA stapling device (US Surgical Corporation). In the left upper quadrant a 5 mm trocar is placed to facilitate entry of the Babcock or grasping device, and in the left lower

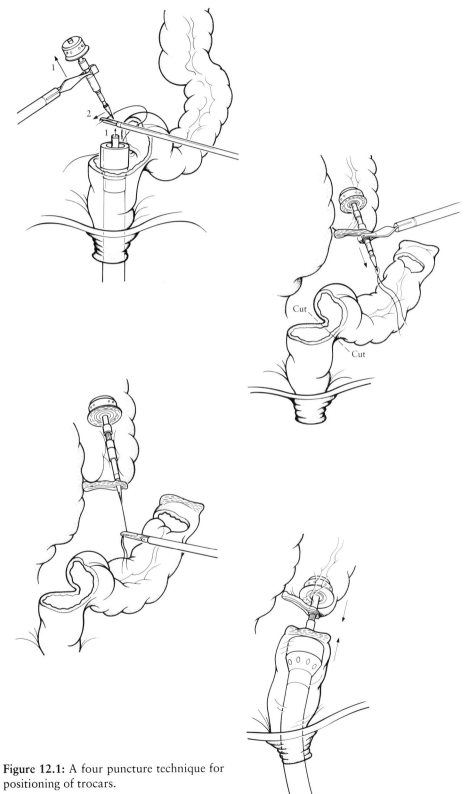

Figure 12.1: A four puncture technique for positioning of trocars.

quadrant a further 10 mm trocar is inserted to allow entry of the telescope for transillumination.

Procedure

A Surgi-needle or Verres needle is inserted into the abdominal cavity, using the usual drop test to make sure that it is placed in the free peritoneal space. Carbon dioxide is insufflated (2.5–3 l) and intra-abdominal pressure is maintained at or below 15 mmHg. A 10 mm telescope is introduced in the right upper quadrant and through this the telescope lens is introduced. An exact inspection of the abdominal cavity is achieved, including examination of the liver, spleen, small intestine and colon. The small intestine is then removed from the pelvis using a hand-over-hand technique as in conventional surgery except that atraumatic graspers are used. In some cases, it is necessary to increase the degree of Trendelenberg to facilitate retention of the small intestine in the upper quadrant of the abdominal cavity.

In a female, the uterus is suspended by inserting a long straight needle percutaneously. This is placed through the fundus of the uterus and brought to the anterior abdominal skin surface where it is clipped loosely using a Kelly or Mosquito clamp. The distal segment of the rectum is identified. A sigmoidoscope is placed in the rectum and, by a process of transillumination, the lesion is identified by decreasing the light intensity of the receptor camera. The operator then puts an endoclip through the right lower quadrant and marks the area of the lesion approximately 3 cm below the transilluminated site. This allows precise determination of the area of resection and the resection margins.

Once the areas of demarcation have been marked with three endoclips, the intestine is suspended by adopting a similar procedure of percutaneously inserting a needle through the abdominal cavity. This is put through the mesentery beneath the colon and then passed to the anterior abdominal wall. Again, this is loosely clipped with a Mosquito clamp on the anterior abdominal wall, care being taken to avoid any sudden traction upon this which may cause damage to the intestine. This step, as can be appreciated, is an improvization.

A similar process can be performed using the endohernia staplers to suspend the intestine from the anterior abdominal wall. The site of suspension which gives the best result in low anterior resections is 2 cm above the peritoneal reflection.

By exerting continuous countertraction, the assistant will move the intestine to the right of the patient to create a cleavage plane. The common iliac vessels and the ureter must be identified. The ureter is traced proximally and distally, and it must be freely available for inspection throughout the abdominal procedure. The dissection is continued proximally along the paracolic gutter on the left side. When using monopolar electrocautery, the power should be reduced by sharp coagulation followed by sharp dissection; this way a safer result can be achieved. It is essential to divide and mobilize the splenicflexure, because additional mobility is required to remove the bowel through the abdominal wall.

The assistant then suspends the intestine to the left side of the patient. This exposes the peritoneum overlying the mesenteric arcade. The right ureter is identified, descending to the pelvis over the common iliac vessels. The demarcation line overlying the right ureter is scored using light cautery. The peritoneum is divided from the root of the mesentery to the pelvic floor, traversing anteriorly to the sigmoid colon, taking care to avoid damage to the bladder. Once the peritoneum has been divided using blunt dissection and light coagulation, the minor vessels of the mesenteric arcade are ligated and divided. The vessels larger than 1.5 mm should be clipped. Smaller vessels can be coagulated either with monopolar or bipolar coagulation or with laser. The use of aqua-dissection is useful in these cases; this helps to raise the peritoneum and free it from the underlying mesenteric fat and vasculature.

Transillumination

Once the peritoneum and the fatty tissue have been skeletonized to a large extent, the transilluminating telescope or lens can be introduced in the left lower quadrant. The light intensity on the receptor camera is reduced and the vasculature can be demarcated. The most useful way of dividing and creating windows in the mesentery is to use a laser with a HE–NE beam which allows the operator to guide his instrument through the darkness of transillumination. Windows are created to the margin of the intestine.

The vasculature is skeletonized to facilitate the application of the titanium clips. The skeletonization is continued to the margin of the intestine. An EndoGIA stapling device is introduced through the right lower quadrant 12 mm port. This is placed across the distal margin of resection of the intestine. The cartridge size is determined by applying an endogauge to the colon. This will indicate whether a 3.5 mm or 2.5 mm staple leg length is necessary to transect the intestine haemostatically. The GIA is closed and fired and the intestine is transected. It is usual to apply a second stapling device to transect the intestine completely.

The now mobile proximal segment of bowel is elevated to the anterior abdominal wall, placing tension upon the mesenteric arcade. The branches of the mesenteric arteries are skeletonized and ligated with titanium clips. In cases of carcinoma, it is imperative to ligate the inferior mesenteric artery, preferably before mobilization of the entire colon.

In cases of carcinoma, a double stapling technique is employed whereby the proximal segment of the descending colon is transected in a similar fashion with the GIA. This helps to reduce the theoretical possibility of sequestration of carcinoma cells in the proximal bowel. The immobilized and resected specimen of colon is placed in the pelvis to prevent it being obscured by the overlying loops of intestine. The proximal staple line is grasped by an atraumatic grasping forceps and brought to the left lower quadrant 10 mm port site. The skin incision is continued immediately to 2.5 cm. The fascia is divided and a muscle split incision is achieved. The incision must be large enough to allow the easy introduction of the anvil head and to remove the specimen.

The mobilized segment of bowel is exteriorized, a purse string applier (US Surgical Corporation) is applied to the proximal portion of bowel and the jaws are closed. The excess intestine is excised and a sizer is introduced into the bowel to determine which size anvil head will be used to fashion the anastomosis. The purse string is tightened with inversion of the intestine snugly on the shaft of the anvil. The anvil and intestine are reintroduced into the peritoneal cavity and placed in the pelvis. A purse string prolene suture is applied to the peritoneum and fascia and the 10 mm trocar is introduced into this defect. The new pneumoperitoneum is recreated, the distal resected specimen of intestine is grasped with a grasping forceps and brought to the left-sided incision site, and removed from the abdominal cavity.

In cases of serosal involvement, an impermeable bag is introduced into the abdomen and the specimen is placed in this. After the tumour specimen has been removed, the trocar is also removed from the abdominal cavity and the fascia and skin are closed on the left lower quadrant.

Specially devised grasping forceps are introduced into the right lower quadrant to grasp the anvil of the stapling device. This is now placed adjacent to the rectal stump.

The assistant surgeon places the PCEEA through the anus and advances the trocar 1 mm to the side of the staple line. After penetration of the rectal stump the trocar is removed with the grasping forceps through the 12 mm port. The grasping device is reintroduced into the abdominal cavity to grasp the anvil shaft and this is coupled to the locking mechanism on the circular stapler introduced through the rectum. The anvil is closed snugly as indicated by the stapling device. The locking mechanism is unlocked and the staples are fired. The anastomosis is fashioned. The stapling mechanism is opened and twisted two turns and then removed from the rectum. Saline is insufflated into the abdominal cavity and, using a colonoscope, air is insufflated into the rectum to reveal any leaks from the anastomotic line. Excellent visualization of the anastomotic line is achieved with the colonoscope to identify and examine the anastomotic line.

A drain is placed only in cases of purulent inflammatory bowel disease or where excessive dissection is performed. There is a final inspection of the mesenteric defect and areas of dissection to determine whether there is any residual bleeding, and finally irrigation of the abdominal cavity is achieved using a pulsed irrigation system (Davol). The trocars are removed after decompression of the abdominal cavity and the wounds are closed with a 30 maxon subcuticular stitch.

Suggested further reading

1   Dubois F, Icard P, Berthelot G and Levard H (1990) Coelioscopic cholecystectomy. Preliminary report of 35 cases. *Ann. Surg.* **211**:60–2.

2   Leahy PF (1989) Technique of laparoscopic appendicectomy. *Br. J. Surg.* **76**:616.

3   Palmer R and Imendioff M (1962) La Place de coelioscopie dans le diagnostic et le traitement des sterilities et des grosses ectopiques. *Rev. Fr. Gynaecol.* **42**:113.

4   Reddick EJ, Olsen DO, Daniell JF, Sayo WB, *et al.* (1989) Laparoscopic laser cholecystectomy. *Laser Med. Surg. News.* **7**:38–40.

5   Semm K (1988) Die Pelviskopische Appendektomie. *Dtsh. Med. Wschr.* **113**:3–5.

6   Zakharova GN and Berthelot G (1989) Laparoscopy in the diagnosis of acute appendicitis in children. *Vestn. Khir.* **141**(12):45–8.

References

Cooperman AN, Katz V, Zimmon D and Botero G (1991) Laparoscopic colon resection: A case report. *J. Laparoendosc. Surg.* **1**:221–4.

Fowler DL and White SA (1991) Laparoscopy assisted sigmoid resection. *Surg. Laparosc. Endosc.* **1**:183–8.

Jacobs M, Verdeja JC and Goldstein HS (1991) Minimally invasive colon resection. *Surg. Laparosc. Endosc.* **1**:144–50.

Peters WR and Bartels TL (1993) Minimally invasive colectomy: Are the potential benefits realised? *Dis. Colon Rectum.*

13

Laparoscopy for the Acute Abdomen

HUMPHREY J. SCOTT

In the acute abdomen, taking a thorough history, performing a thorough clinical examination and excluding medical causes have long remained the mainstays of management. Zachary Cope, a surgeon at St Mary's Hospital, London, finished his classic book *The diagnosis of the acute abdomen in rhyme*[1]:

> *In doubtful cases do not wait too long*
> *Before exploring for it is quite wrong*
> *To act upon the slogan Wait and See*
> *When looking might provide the remedy.*

When Sir Zachary Cope composed the above lines, 'looking' was considered to imply a diagnostic laparotomy. The advice still holds good today, although a 'diagnostic laparoscopy' may provide the remedy.

The aim of a diagnostic laparoscopy is to achieve a diagnosis with as little insult on the patient as is possible. The recovery time and hospital stay after a diagnostic laparoscopy are considerably shorter than after a diagnostic laparotomy. The surgeon also benefits, as the complication rate is lower after a laparoscopy than a laparotomy. The surgeon's activity remains unaffected (although it could possibly be increased with laparoscopy being performed on cases he would previously have observed for a longer duration) and the bed occupancy figures improve accordingly. The provider and purchaser benefits as the overall cost is reduced (*see* Figure 13.1).

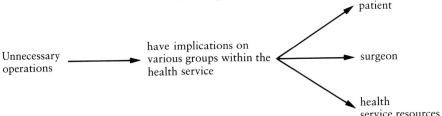

Figure 13.1: Diagram showing the implications of unnecessary operations.

Although laparoscopy has been well known for over 80 years – it was described by Ruddock[2] in 1937 for peritoneoscopy, and by Gazzaniga[3] and Carnevale[4] in the 1970s for abdominal trauma – it remains a specialized technique for the acute abdomen, practised in only a few centres in the UK.

Before the introduction of the microchip camera and television screen, emergency laparoscopy was confined almost solely to gynaecologists. There were not many operating rooms where a general surgeon and gynaecologist operated together with a laparoscope on a patient with an acute abdomen of unknown aetiology. This was probably due to the historical practice of patients being admitted to hospital under one consultant who is responsible for their management. Shared care is unusual with patients admitted through accident and emergency departments, and it is often difficult for the general surgeon and gynaecologist on duty to find a mutually agreeable time to take a patient to theatre. Thus laparoscopy remained under the auspices of gynaecologists who summoned general surgeons, if required, after they had attained a laparoscopic diagnosis.

The introduction of laparoscopic equipment into general surgical operating theatres has followed the development of laparoscopic cholecystectomy. Consultants may learn slowly at first but, as their expertise gathers pace, they pass on their knowledge to their junior staff. The use of the laparoscope in diagnosis and management of the acute abdomen is slowly growing in the UK.

With the introduction of endoscopic surgery, laparoscopy also has an ever-increasing role in the definitive operative treatment in the acute abdomen. The remainder of this chapter is divided into two parts, dealing first with laparoscopy as a diagnostic tool, and then with operative laparoscopy for conditions presenting with an acute abdomen.

Laparoscopy as a diagnostic tool in the general surgeon's armamentarium

A detailed and thorough history and physical examination (with or without resuscitation) should remain the first line of management for the acute abdomen. Several well-established routine investigations have been added to the clinical assessment. These include the presence of fever, urine microscopy and the results of serum amylase and white cell count. However, none of these investigations have convincingly contributed to the sensitivity or specificity of a diagnosis[5], although leucocytosis has been shown to be of value in determining the diagnosis of appendicitis in the first 48 hours following admission[6].

Laparoscopy must be seen in the context of the other diagnostic aids which have been thoroughly reviewed[5,12] and are available to the surgeon:

1. Computer-aided diagnosis (CAD)

The CAD computer uses formalized bayesian probabilities based on a large database of previous associations, whereas a clinician uses his previous experience and acquired knowledge. When introduced to clinical practice, CAD has reduced the negative laparotomy rate to 10%[7]. Although CAD has been shown to help attain a diagnosis, it is not readily available in clinical practice. This could be due to:

- clinicians refusing to use computers in patient management

- a high rate of 'non-specific abdominal pain' diagnoses reached in several series

- the fact that laparoscopy has been shown to give results that are as good as those obtained by CAD, with the additional advantage that it provides a precise diagnosis on which non-operative management can be based[8].

2. Ultrasonography

Ultrasound scanning has been used for many years for hepatobiliary problems as it is a highly sensitive and specific test for gallstones. It is being increasingly used in the assessment of acute and chronic abdomens as it is non-invasive and has few side-effects. Diagnostic accuracy is related to the expertise of the ultrasonographer. This technique has shown a 75% sensitivity with a 100% specificity for appendicitis in The Netherlands[9]. There are, however, few hospitals where the required expertise for abdominal ultrasonography is reliably available outside normal working hours.

3. Plain and contrast radiography

Plain abdominal radiographs have been shown to influence patient management in only 4% of cases. An additional erect abdominal film is of little value, although an erect chest radiograph is useful in detecting free abdominal gas.

In the acute abdomen situation, upper gastrointestinal contrast studies using water-soluble material are useful in detecting oesophageal and peptic perforation. In a study from Hong Kong, this technique was used to attain the diagnosis of perforated peptic ulcer prior to aggressive conservative treatment[10]. Water-soluble contrast enemas have a definite role in identifying a leak in acute diverticulitis and aiding the management and diagnosis of patients with large bowel obstruction.

4. White cell scanning

This technique commonly uses radiolabelled indium or ^{99m}Technetium hexamethyl propylene amine oxime white cells. In addition to a gamma camera and labelling facilities, it also requires 12–24 hours for adequate imaging of areas of concentrated white cells. The time and expertise required limit its use in the acute abdomen.

5. Fine catheter aspiration

Peritoneal lavage, either through a subumbilical or four quadrant tap, is commonly used for assessment of the acute abdomen in blunt trauma. Although it improves the diagnosis of intra-abdominal bleeding, not every positive test requires laparotomy, as the bleeding may have stopped spontaneously or may have been caused by insertion of the catheter.

Fine catheter aspiration and peritoneal cytology have been shown to improve clinical decision-making by measuring the proportion of polymorphonuclear cells in the aspirate[11] of acute abdomens. However, the specimens were stained by a modified Romanowsky method and a cytologist's expertise was used. This technique is not widely used and appears to remain an experimental tool.

Laparoscopy is more invasive than any of the above techniques and most surgeons perform it under general anaesthetic. However, a study from Leeds in 1980 reported the value of laparoscopy under local anaesthesia in 250 medical and surgical patients[13]. Only nine patients were recorded as having an acute abdomen, and all patients apparently tolerated the procedure well. Laparoscopy for acute abdominal pain was first described as a preoperative procedure 17 years ago[14]. Since then, studies have looked at the role of laparoscopy in decision-making in patients presenting with right iliac fossa and pelvic pain. A selective policy of laparoscopy, taken as a part of the overall clinical decision-making process, has been shown to improve diagnostic and patient outcome results. Management error in a group of patients with acute abdominal pain, in whom the decision to operate was in doubt, reduced from 19% to 0%[15].

A study from Vancouver reported on the introduction and application of laparoscopy in a general abdominal surgeon's practice[16]. In consecutive cases, laparoscopy was shown to have a 90% diagnostic accuracy in the acute abdomen. In 17 patients (55%), laparotomy was avoided because another cause of the acute abdomen was identified. A large proportion of these cases were gynaecological.

The indications for diagnostic laparoscopy are the same as those for diagnostic laparotomy, with some important exclusions: pregnancy; children, where small laparoscopes are unavailable; small or large bowel obstruction; and in cases where there is a high risk of causing a iatrogenic injury (such as bowel perforation or carbon dioxide embolus) due to the laparoscopic procedure. In these cases, an open procedure is indicated.

The technique for diagnostic laparoscopy is identical to any other laparoscopic procedure. In cases of abdominal stabbing, the stab wound should be closed with suture material or sealed with elastoplast for the duration of the procedure. The bladder is usually emptied or the patient is asked to void prior to theatre. Insufflation with carbon dioxide is achieved using a Verres needle through a subumbilical incision. The laparoscope is introduced through the subumbilical incision.

The abdomen should be systematically examined in all four quadrants, the pelvis and around the subhepatic spaces. Further 5 mm trocars may be introduced under direct vision to allow the passage of cannulae, grasping forceps and other instruments. These can manipulate, provide suction, retract, coagulate and help in peritoneoscopy.

At the end of this procedure, the operator should have a clear idea of his next management step, which might be to:

- convert to an open procedure

- attempt a laparoscopic procedure and convert if necessary

- instigate medical treatment

- continue a period of observation.

The next part of this chapter examines laparoscopic procedures which may be performed after a laparoscopic diagnosis has been made.

Laparoscopic operations in the acute abdomen

Appendicectomy

Until a few years ago, the selection of patients to be laparoscoped prior to the open operation was a matter for debate, as it is well known that up to 30% of open appendicectomies have normal histology. It was generally agreed that young women with an established diagnosis of appendicitis and patients with no definite diagnosis should be laparoscoped[17,18]. Seventeen years ago a study[19] of 223 laparoscopies for acute pelvic pain in women revealed that laparoscopy supported the clinical diagnosis in only 25% of cases, and that laparotomy was avoided in 65% (145 patients). However, the diagnosis of acute appendicitis was confirmed by laparoscopy in only eight of 35 cases admitted with the diagnosis. This low proportion (15.7%) of cases with a preoperative diagnosis of appendicitis probably reflects the fact that the work is from a department of obstetrics and gynaecology where the majority of cases admitted had a preoperative diagnosis of tubal pregnancy.

Today, with the advent of endoscopic surgery, the question being asked is whether all patients with acute abdomens should be laparoscoped and, if appendicitis is confirmed as the diagnosis, should it be removed laparoscopically? The two parts to this question are interwoven because, if patients undergoing laparoscopic appendicectomy have less morbidity, as has been suggested, it follows that all acute abdomens should be laparoscoped.

Early reports suggest that there is improved cosmesis as laparoscopic surgery does not require extension of the incision to mobilize the appendix in difficult cases. It has also been suggested that there is a reduction in wound pain, a shortened hospital stay and quicker return to normal life[20,21]. Evidence is emerging that there may be reduced development of adhesions[22], although long-term follow-up studies are required.

The two main criticisms of laparoscopic appendicectomy and other laparoscopic operations for the acute abdomen are that they cost too much and take too long. The cost of a laparoscopic appendicectomy using modern technology and instruments (which will soon be readily available in most hospitals) will be counterbalanced by the advantages conferred on the patient as discussed above. The time for the diagnostic laparoscopy and laparoscopic appendicectomy is almost the same as for the open operation in skilled hands[20]. With modern time-saving instruments, and the increasingly rapid acquisition of laparoscopic skills, we may see laparoscopic appendicectomy becoming the operation of choice in the future.

Complicated descriptions and diagrams have been published[23] which appear to deter rather than encourage the general surgeon performing this relatively easy and worthwhile technique.

The standard technique, shown in Figures 13.2 to 13.4, is carried out with a 10 mm laparoscope port introduced subumbilically or in the midepigastric region if the laparoscope and sheath are too close to the appendix in the former position. I use one 5 mm port in the left iliac fossa and one 10 mm port in the right hypochondrium through which the endoloop and endoclips are introduced. The appendix is usually removed through this port.

After insufflation and mobilization of the appendix, the mesentery and the appendicular artery are carefully divided between endoclips up to the base of the appendix (*see* Figure 13.2). The endoloop is passed over the appendix (*see* Figure 13.3). It is tightened (*see* Figure 13.4) and the appendix is divided with diathermy scissors distal to the endoloop. Some surgeons diathermy the appendix stump. The appendix and its attached mesentery are removed.

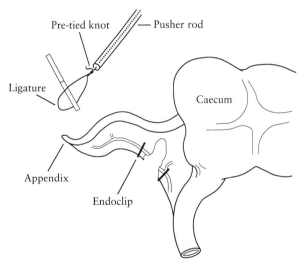

Figure 13.2: After insufflation and mobilization of the appendix, the mesentery and the appendicular artery are carefully divided between endoclips up to the base of the appendix.

I have modified this technique. After mobilizing the appendix, I make a small hole in the appendix mesentery at the junction at the base of the appendix (*see* Figure 13.5). Three endoclips clip the base of the appendix using the defect in the mesentery (*see* Figure 13.6). The appendix is divided between endoclips,

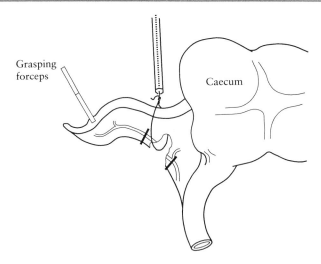

Figure 13.3: The endoloop is passed over the appendix.

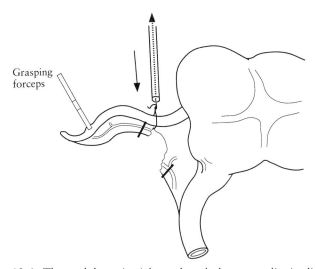

Figure 13.4: The endoloop is tightened and the appendix is divided with diathermy scissors distal to the endoloop.

leaving two on the stump (*see* Figure 13.7). The appendix is removed from its mesentery using a hook diathermy running up beside the appendix (*see* Figure 13.8). The appendix is removed through the right hypogastric port.

There appear to be four advantages using the latter technique. The endoclip application is quick and accurate. There is very little bleeding as only the terminal branches of the appendicular artery are coagulated, whereas in the former technique the main trunk of the artery is divided between endoclips. Neither technique describes burial of the appendix stump; however, by leaving the majority of the appendicular mesentery behind, it can act as an 'omentum' and cover the stump. In addition, removal of the appendix through an anterior abdominal wall port is facilitated as there is no attached mesentery.

New techniques are being described[24], which involve delivering the appen-

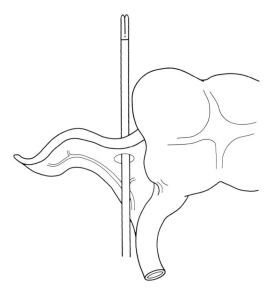

Figure 13.5: In a modification of the technique where the appendix stump is diathermied, a small hole is made in the appendix mesentery at the junction of the base of the appendix.

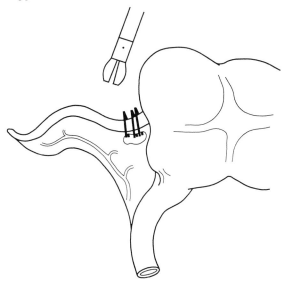

Figure 13.6: Three endoclips clip the base of the appendix using the defect in the mesentery.

dix and base of caecum through a 12 mm port placed at McBurney's point. The appendix and its mesentery are ligated and divided. The base of the caecum is returned to the abdominal cavity.

As with most laparoscopic operations, new techniques and methods will undoubtedly continue to be described.

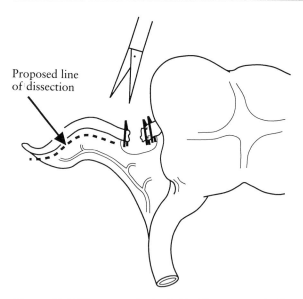

Proposed line
of dissection

Figure 13.7: The appendix is divided between endoclips, leaving two on the stump.

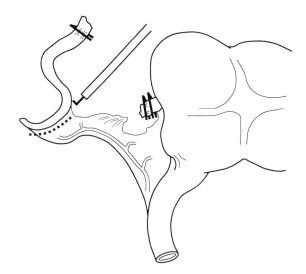

Figure 13.8: The appendix is removed from its mesentery using a hook diathermy running up beside the appendix.

Blunt trauma

Urgent laparoscopy can reduce the number of unnecessary abdominal explorations in injured patients following blunt abdominal trauma. The technique can be performed in the accident and emergency department or the intensive care unit, as well as in theatre. It can easily be performed under local anaesthetic. The role of peritoneal lavage, which requires the same amount of anaesthesia, has been discussed earlier in this chapter.

Berci and colleagues[26] describe the technique, applying 1% lidocaine to the midline and performing the insufflation and laparoscopy through a subumbilical incision. An additional right or left upper lateral quadrant port can be fashioned under direct vision, after injecting the site with local anaesthetic, if abdominal content manipulation, retraction, suction or coagulation is required. The importance of systematic examination, including all quadrants, the pelvis and the supra-hepatic spaces, is emphasized.

Laparoscopy's obvious advantage over peritoneal lavage is that the distribution of the blood can provide a clue to the location of the bleeding site, ie around the liver, in the left hypochondrium around the spleen or in the pelvis. The amount of bleeding is difficult to quantify laparoscopically, but has been divided[26] into minimal, moderate and severe.

Minimal. This is where there is a small amount of blood in the lateral gutters or where streaks of blood are found between the intestinal loops. The actual bleeding site is often not found but, if the volume of blood appears unchanged, the patient can usually be observed. Small volumes of blood can provide a positive lavage.

Moderate. A 5–10 mm deep blood level is seen in the paracolic gutters. A second trocar can be introduced and the haemoperitoneum evacuated with suction. A search for the bleeding point can be made, using the suction cannula as a retractor. If the bleeding site is identified, appropriate action can be taken: either by laparoscopically coagulating and suturing the bleeding point and applying an alginate sealant if necessary, or by performing open surgery with an incision above the source of haemorrhage. The laparoscopy allows the surgeon to select the optimal incision. If, after 5–10 minutes' searching, the bleeding point has not been identified, and a haemoperitoneum has recollected in the paracolic gutters, the source of the haemorrhage is probably not within visualization of the laparoscope. A formal open laparotomy is therefore indicated.

Severe. The cardiovascular status of the patient may preclude laparoscopy in this situation, and open laparotomy may be performed on clinical indications alone. However, if a pneumoperitoneum is created and large pools of blood are seen, the indication for immediate operation is obvious.

A 25-year-old woman was admitted 48 hours after a road traffic accident in which she had fallen off her bicycle onto her right-hand side. She had suffered no loss of consciousness and was assessed at an accident and emergency department near the site of the fall. She had been discharged and was told to seek medical advice if she became symptomatic. She presented at our accident and emergency department complaining of right hypochondrial pain and right shoulder tip pain. She was haemodynamically stable and there was no obvious abnormality on physical examination other than mild tenderness and guarding in the right hypochondrium. She had a mild leucocytosis and it was decided to perform a diagnostic laparoscopy.

A small amount of free bile was seen around the liver. This was aspirated, and using the suction cannula as a retractor, the liver and bowel were examined. No liver tear was visualized and the bile ducts and gallbladder appeared intact. No other abnormality was seen. A drain was inserted; this drained 50 ml of bile over 24 hours and then stopped. She experienced no further abdominal or shoulder tip pain after the laparoscopy and was discharged on the third day. She remains well one year after the incident.

This case demonstrates how laparoscopy can successfully treat and reduce the operative stay in patients who present with blunt trauma.

Perforated duodenal ulcer

Although the diagnosis may be suspected preoperatively, laparoscopy affords the surgeon the opportunity to confirm his clinical diagnosis. Bile-stained fluid may be seen in the paracolic gutters and around the porta hepatis. Omentum overlying the duodenum may have to be gently removed in order to visualize the perforation.

Laparoscopic oversew can be performed in an identical way to the open method. Thorough washout can be clearly visualized, and the advantages of performing this urgent surgery with minimal access techniques are the same as those for any other laparoscopic operation.

Penetrating injuries

A 37-year-old man was admitted after being stabbed with a knife in his left iliac fossa. The passage of radio-opaque material down the stab wound confirmed entry into the peritoneal cavity. As he had a rigid, quiet abdomen, laparoscopy was performed. The entry site was temporarily sealed. Routing insufflation and laparoscopy through a subumbilical incision was performed. The entry site into the peritoneal cavity was observed. There was no haemoperitoneum, serosal tear or peritoneal soiling. He was discharged on the third day. If he had undergone an open laparotomy, his hospital stay would have been longer.

Along with other authors[26], we do not advocate laparoscopy for gunshot wounds but recommend its use for other types of penetrating trauma.

Other procedures

Laparoscopy and endoscopic surgery are finding many new uses in the acute abdomen. Laparoscopic fixation of a sigmoid volvulus has been described[27], and we have excised torted fimbrial cysts laparoscopically in women presenting with right iliac fossa pain. No doubt further procedures and techniques will be developed.

Training

Patients presenting with an acute abdomen may provide the best way for junior staff, under appropriate supervision, to learn the basic insufflation techniques, become used to handling the laparoscope and camera, become oriented in the peritoneum and perform simple operative techniques. Laparoscopy in the acute abdomen will not only benefit the patient, it will also benefit many trainee surgeons who will be introduced to this general surgical adjunct this way.

Acknowledgement: I wish to thank Mr Alan Dedman, Audio-Visual Services Department, St Mary's Hospital, London, for his help with the illustrations.

References

1   Cope VZ (1947) *The diagnosis of the acute abdomen in rhyme* (by Zeta). H.K. Lewis, London.

2   Ruddock JC (1937) Peritoneoscopy. *Surg. Gynecol. Obstet.* **65**:523–39.

3   Gazzaniga AB, Slanton WW and Bartlett RH (1976) Laparoscopy in the diagnosis of blunt and penetrating injuries to the abdomen. *Am. J. Surg.* **131**:315–18.

4   Carnevale N, Baron N and Delany HM (1977) Peritoneoscopy as an aid in the diagnosis of abdominal trauma: a preliminary report. *J. Trauma.* **17**:634–41.

5   Paterson-Brown S (1991) Strategies for reducing inappropriate laparotomy rate in the acute abdomen. *Br. Med. J.* **303**:1115–18.

6   McCombe AW and Gunn AA (1991) Laparotomy and the acute abdomen. *Br. Med. J.* **303**:1476.

7   Adams ID, Chan M and Clifford P *et al.* (1986) Computer aided diagnosis of acute abdominal pain: a multicentre study. *Br. Med. J.* **293**:800–4.

8   Paterson-Brown S, Vipond MN and Simms K *et al.* (1989) Clinical decision-making and laparoscopy versus computer prediction in the management of the acute abdomen. *Br. J. Surg.* **76**:1011–13.

9   Puyaert JBCM, Rutgers PH and Lalisang RI *et al.* (1987) A prospective study of ultrasonography in the diagnosis of acute appendicitis. *N. Engl. J. Med.* **317**:666–9.

10 Crofts TJ, Park KGM and Steele RJC *et al.* (1989) A randomized trial of nonoperative treatment for perforated peptic ulcer. *N. Engl. J. Med.* **320**:970–3.

11 Vipond MN, Paterson-Brown S and Tyrell MR *et al.* (1990) Evaluation of fine catheter aspiration cytology of the peritoneum as an adjunct to decision making in the acute abdomen. *Br. J. Surg.* **77**:86–7.

12 Paterson-Brown S and Vipond MN (1990) Modern aids to clinical decision-making in the acute abdomen. *Br. J. Surg.* **77**:13–18.

13 Hall TJ, Donaldson DR and Brennan TG (1980) The value of laparoscopy under local anaesthesia in 250 medical and surgical patients. *Br. J. Surg.* **67**:751–3.

14 Sugarbaker PH, Bloom BS, Sanders JH and Wilson RE (1975) Preoperative laparoscopy in diagnosis of acute abdominal pain. *Lancet*. i:442–5.

15 Paterson-Brown S, Eckersley JRT, Sim AJW and Dudley HAF (1986) Laparoscopy as an adjunct to decision-making in the 'acute abdomen'. *Br. J. Surg*. 73:1022–24.

16 Nagy AG and James D (1989) Diagnostic laparoscopy. *Am. J. Surg*. 157:490–3.

17 Foster H McA (1988) Which patients should undergo laparoscopy? *Br. Med. J*. 297:489.

18 Deutsch AA, Zelikovsky A and Reiss R (1982) Laparoscopy in the prevention of unnecessary appendicectomies: a prospective study. *Br. J. Surg*. 69:336–7.

19 Anteby SO, Schenker JG and Polishuk WZ (1975) The value of laparoscopy in acute pelvic pain. *Ann. Surg*. 181:484–6.

20 Loh A and Taylor RS (1992) Laparoscopic appendicectomy. *Br. J. Surg*. 79:289–90.

21 Austin O, Hederman WP and O'Connell PR *et al*. (1992) *Prospective evaluation of laparoscopic versus open appendicectomy*. Presentation to the Association of Surgeons of Great Britain and Ireland, Jersey, April.

22 de Wilde RL (1991) Goodbye to late bowel obstruction after appendicectomy. *Lancet*. 338:1012.

23 Tate J (1992) Introduction to laparoscopic surgical techniques: part 2. *Hospital Update*. 18:19–24.

24 Byrne DS, Bell G, Morrice JJ and Orr G (1992) Technique for laparoscopic appendicectomy. *Br. J. Surg*. 79:574–5.

26 Berci G, Sackier JM and Paz-Partlow M (1991) Emergency laparoscopy. *Am. J. Surg*. 161:332–5.

27 Miller R, Roe AM, Eltingham WK and Espiner HJ (1992) Laparoscopic fixation of sigmoid volvulus. *Br. J. Surg*. 79:435.

14

Laparoscopic Surgical Treatment of Peptic Ulcer Disease

NAMIR KATKHOUDA, JEAN MOUIEL AND STEPHEN WHITE

Laparoscopic surgery provides efficient treatment for both elective and emergency duodenal ulceration[1]. There is now universal agreement about the advantages of minimal access surgery to patients in terms of fewer days in hospital, quicker return to work and improved quality of life.

The natural history of duodenal ulcer is of life-long recurrent symptoms with eventual complications in 20% of patients, eg bleeding, stenosis or perforation. Long-term medical therapy is the option currently offered to most patients; however, side-effects are common, compliance is poor and surveillance and medication are expensive. Furthermore, since the introduction of H_2 blockers 20 years ago, the mortality of peptic ulcer has not decreased but has actually increased, for example in the UK[2,3]. Patients and doctors should unfortunately regard duodenal ulcer as a life-long disease.

Our results with laparoscopic vagotomy for duodenal ulcer will encourage gastroenterologists and surgeons to inform their patients of what is now state-of-the-art treatment. However, maintaining today's excellent results and avoiding the postoperative problems of open vagotomy will require an experienced surgeon with an enthusiastic team, aided by optimal equipment.

Laparoscopic operation for duodenal ulcer was first performed at Hospital St Roch in 1989[4]. Since then the procedures described have been repeated in selected centres worldwide with minimum reported morbidity. The current range of operations includes:

- posterior truncal vagotomy and anterior seromyotomy

- posterior truncal vagotomy and anterior highly selective vagotomy

- complete truncal vagotomy

- patching of perforation and anti-ulcer operation.

In this institution, the Taylor procedure (posterior truncal vagotomy and anterior seromyotomy) is currently the preferred elective treatment for duodenal ulcer, as it is simple, reproducible and efficient. The future advances in laparoscopic instrument design should ensure that surgeons are soon performing gastric bypass, gastric resection and gastric reconstruction for other complications of gastroduodenal peptic ulceration.

Selection of the patient

The preoperative evaluation of patients with duodenal ulcer is the same as in traditional open surgery. The investigation includes physical examination and routine biochemical screening to exclude other systemic disorders. Contraindications to laparoscopy, both relative and absolute, are the same as those described for cholecystectomy.

Any patient with recurrent ulcer symptoms and an unhealed ulcer after two years of full compliance with medical therapy should be considered a candidate for elective surgery. It may be of benefit to those patients with duodenal ulcer who regularly use ulcerogenic medication (such as NSAIDs and aspirin) or who drink alcohol or smoke excessively, to be referred for surgery earlier. Anaemia or repeated minor bleeding should also warrant surgical intervention in under two years.

Endoscopy should be performed to visualize the area of disease directly to determine if duodenal stenosis has occurred. Biopsies should be sent to exclude the organism *Helicobacter pylori* and other rare causes of duodenal ulceration, eg Crohn's disease. In addition, endoscopy excludes other diseases of the upper gastrointestinal tract (gastric carcinoma, gastro-oesophageal reflux, etc) in which symptoms may mimic those of peptic ulcer disease.

Secretory studies are useful to demonstrate a postoperative reduction of acid output and to provide a means to assess the effectiveness of the vagotomy. Measurement of basal acid output (BAO) and peak acid output (PAO) following pentagastrin (6 μg/kg) will show marked hyperacidity in most duodenal ulcer patients.

Selection of the operation

This choice will reflect the experience and training of the surgeon, together with details of the patient's ulcer.

The Taylor procedure (posterior truncal vagotomy and anterior sero-myotomy) has proved equal to other selective vagotomies in the healing of duodenal ulcer. Taylor *et al.*[5] reported only a 6% incidence of recurrent ulceration at the fifth year of follow-up in his personal series. Other reports of the Taylor procedure[6,7] indicate five year recurrence ulcer rates of 14% and 12% respectively. The operation is considerably easier than highly selective vagotomy in obese patients, and obviously involves diminished risk of damage to the nerve of Latarjet and of ischaemic necrosis of the lesser curve.

Posterior truncal vagotomy and anterior highly selective vagotomy, first reported in 1991[8], is based on an operation originally described in 1978[9].

Unfortunately, no other studies in open surgery are available to assess the efficacy of this procedure.

Complete truncal vagotomy achieves ulcer healing in 99% of patients; however, because of unavoidable pyloric spasm and gastric stasis, 15–25% require pyloric dilatation. Postoperatively this latter procedure has a high failure rate. The experience with this procedure is limited, although Dubois continues to use it in selected patients where ulcer healing cannot be achieved by less radical measures.

Patching/oversew of the duodenal perforation and an anti-ulcer operation should be performed together on all fit patients presenting within 12 hours of chemical peritonitis. However, elderly patients with associated medical diseases, presenting after a delay of 12 hours, should be considered to be at high risk and receive only a simple omental patch of the perforation.

Preparation

As in traditional open surgery, general anaesthesia and endotracheal intubation are advised. We do not routinely insert bladder catheters for upper abdominal laparoscopic procedures. It is more convenient for the patient to void when leaving the ward. Nasogastric aspiration is necessary to ensure that the stomach is empty.

The patient is placed supine with the legs apart in the French position. The surgeon stands between the legs with an assistant on either side. The entire operating room staff should have a direct view of a video screen. The patient is prepared and draped and instruments laid out in case laparotomy should be necessary.

The pneumoperitoneum is established via an umbilical puncture and maintained to a pressure of 14 mmHg using carbon dioxide. The first trocar 10 mm (Ethicon) is inserted 5 cm above and to the right of the umbilicus. A forward-viewing 0° laparoscope (Karl Storz) is inserted and the remaining trocars are introduced under direct vision, as shown in Figure 14.1. A 10 mm trocar is next placed opposite the camera through the left rectus muscle. This

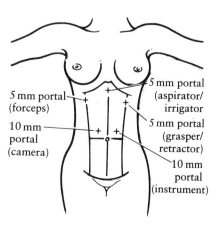

Figure 14.1: Trocar sites.

is the operating channel, through which the hook coagulator, scissors, and clip or staplers are later introduced. 5 mm trocars are inserted subcostally right and left along the mid-clavicular line. Lastly, the xiphoid trocar 5 mm is used for introducing blunt retractors and aspiration/irrigation probes. The abdominal cavity should first be explored to determine that the laparoscopic approach is feasible.

Technique

Taylor's posterior truncal vagotomy and anterior seromyotomy

This selective vagotomy of the stomach achieves parietal cell denervation whilst preserving maximum antral motility. The technique of denervation is based upon anatomical studies which demonstrate how the anterior gastric nerve branches, after reaching the lesser curve, take an oblique passage through the three muscle layers before reaching the submucosal plexus. Taylor[10] thus described dividing these anterior gastric nerves by making a seromuscular incision along the line of the lesser curve, which together with the posterior truncal vagotomy, ensured complete parietal cell denervation. Sufficient antral motility is preserved by the posterior submucosal connections of the anterior nerve of Latarjet[11]. The procedure takes placed in three steps:

- approaching the hiatus

- posterior truncal vagotomy

- anterior seromyotomy.

APPROACHING THE HIATUS
The left lobe of the liver is retracted upwards by the assistant using a blunt probe through the xiphoid port. The lesser omentum is opened high up near the gastro-oesophageal junction via an avascular window (*see* Figure 14.2). A small coronary vein or accessory left hepatic artery may require ligation as this window is enlarged towards the hiatus. Within the lesser sac, peritoneum covering the right crus and abdominal oesophagus is now incised longitudinally over 3–4 cm. The remaining dissection of the hiatus is completed, disturbing as few of the supporting structures as possible.

POSTERIOR TRUNCAL VAGOTOMY
The right crus is now grasped and retracted away from the oesophagus, which can be identified with the aid of nasogastric tube movement. The plane between the oesophagus and right crus is opened to expose the posterior wall and meso-oesophagus. Within the depths of this angle, the white cord of the posterior vagus is easily recognized by its pearly appearance. It is lifted up with the hook and stripped of its vaso vasorum. The nerve is then transected between two clips and sent for histological confirmation (*see* Figure 14.3).

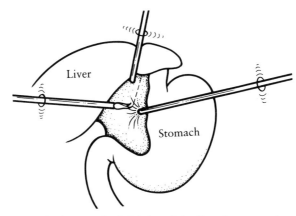

Figure 14.2: Approaching the hiatus, the left lobe of the liver is retracted upwards by the assistant using a blunt probe through the xiphoid port. The lesser omentum is opened high up near the gastro-oesophageal junction via an avascular window.

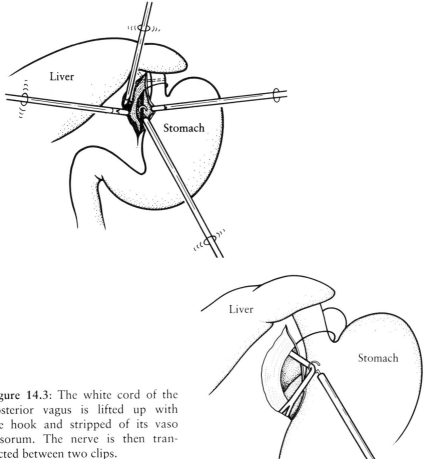

Figure 14.3: The white cord of the posterior vagus is lifted up with the hook and stripped of its vaso vasorum. The nerve is then transected between two clips.

ANTERIOR SEROMYOTOMY

The anterior surface of the stomach is grasped and put on the stretch while the line of seromyotomy is marked with the hook coagulator. The line of incision begins on the cardia at the left angle of the gastro-oesophageal junction and continues exactly 1.5 cm from, and parallel to, the margin of the lesser curvature, stopping 5–7 cm from the pylorus at the level of the crow's foot.

Taylor's original description involved a seromyotomy from only the right side of the gastro-oesophageal junction with a neurectomy across the anterior surface of the oesophagus. However, a simple modification to extend the seromyotomy proximally ensures sectioning the criminal nerve of Grassi and other aberrant branches along the left margin of the oesophagus[12].

Prior to deepening the seromyotomy, three or four large serosal vessels crossing the line will need to be dissected and ligated. This will ensure minimal bleeding as the dissection is deepened.

The hook coagulator is set to half cut/half coag. Grasping forceps apply stretch as the serosa is cut in 2–3 cm lengths. A combination of blunt separation and cutting by the hook, with firm retraction of the cut edges, exposes the mucosa. Individual nerve fibres will be encountered during this process (*see* Figure 14.4).

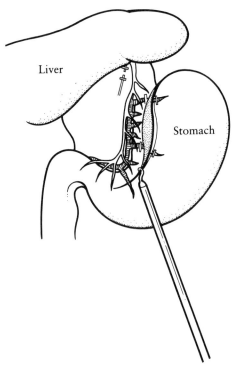

Figure 14.4: Grasping forceps apply stretch and, a combination of blunt separation and cutting by hook, with firm retraction of the cut edges, exposes the mucosa. Individual nerve fibres will be encountered during this process.

The seromyotomy is complete when the mucosa pouts through the muscle cut. The magnification and illumination give the mucosa a recognizable bluish translucency. Occasional submucosal bleeding will require careful coagulation.

To check for perforation, insufflate the stomach and add methylene blue. This procedure should be performed routinely in early cases and for any subsequent doubtful situation. We would recommend repair of any perforation with a two-layered laparoscopic suture, although this has not been necessary in our experience.

The seromyotomy, which now appears as a 10 mm gaping slice, is closed to achieve further haemostasis and reduce adhesions (*see* Figure 14.5A). An overlapping closure is used to prevent nerve regrowth (*see* Figure 14.6). In the past a continuous suture was used; however, more recently the laparoscopic fascial stapler (Ethicon) has been used to reduce operating time (*see* Figure 14.5B).

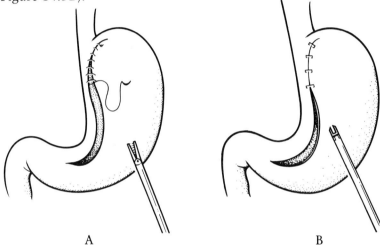

A   B

Figure 14.5A: The seromyotomy, which now appears as a 10 mm gaping slice, is closed to achieve further haemostasis and reduce adhesions. (B) A laparoscopic fascial stapler (Ethicon) is used to reduce operating time.

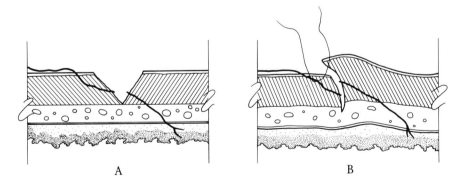

A   B

Figure 14.6: Overlap suture prevents nerve regrowth.

Posterior truncal vagotomy and anterior highly selective vagotomy

This procedure consists of three steps:

- approaching the hiatus

- posterior truncal vagotomy and

- anterior highly selective vagotomy.

The first two steps have already been described.

ANTERIOR HIGHLY SELECTIVE VAGOTOMY
Commence high up on the lesser curve, alongside the abdominal oesophagus where the anterior nerve of Latarjet can be identified. The gastric branches of the anterior vagus are then individually dissected, clipped and ligated as the dissection continues down the lesser curve to the antral crow's foot. Damage to the nerve of Latarjet can be prevented by avoiding excessive handling, diathermy or clipping of the lesser omentum. The operation is complete after the oesophagogastric junction is cleared of the aberrant fundal branches (*see* Figure 14.7).

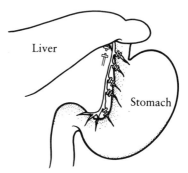

Figure 14.7: Anterior highly selective vagotomy is complete after the oesophagogastric junction is cleared of the aberrant fundal branches.

Complete truncal vagotomy

The procedure consists of four steps:

- approaching the hiatus

- posterior truncal vagotomy

- anterior truncal vagotomy

- pyloric dilatation or gastroenterostomy.

The first two have been previously described.

ANTERIOR TRUNCAL VAGOTOMY
The phreno-oesophageal peritoneum is incised anteriorly over the abdominal oesophagus. The anterior vagus is usually more than a single trunk at this level and special attention should be paid to those aberrant fundal branches along the left side of the oesophagus. With the use of traction and palpation, however, one can 'roll' the oesophagus as in open surgery and expose this left

edge. The clarity and magnification provided by the laparoscope ensure that each nerve branch is dissected free and ligated with minimal disturbance of the oesophageal muscle wall.

PYLORIC DILATATION

The dilatation is performed using a fibre-optic endoscopic balloon during the same operative procedures, although some surgeons choose to perform the procedure postoperatively. After ascertaining the correct position, the balloon is gently inflated under manometric control to 45 psi for 10 minutes[13]. The results of this procedure are unpredictable and may need to be repeated (*see* Figure 14.8).

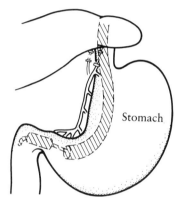

Figure 14.8: For pyloric dilatation the balloon is gently inflated under manometric control to 45 psi for 10 minutes.

LAPAROSCOPIC GASTROENTEROSTOMY

The more reliable method to ensure adequate gastric emptying is to construct a gastric drainage bypass[14]. The first loop of jejunum is anastomosed in an antecolic side to side fashion to the juxtapyloric anterior surface of the stomach. A small 10 mm gastrostomy and enterostomy are made to allow introduction of the two arms of the endoscopic linear cutter. After checking that the posterior and anterior aspects are free, the stapler is fired, removed, reloaded and reinserted. A second cut enlarges the anastomosis to approximately 6 cm. The edges of the gastrostomy and enterostomy are then approximated, after which the defect can be closed and cut clean again with the EndoGIA (*see* Figure 14.9).

Management of perforated duodenal ulcer

Acute duodenal perforations are usually anterior and easily identified through the laparoscope. Initially, only four ports are required (excluding the fifth left subcostal port). The peritoneal contaminant is collected and sent for culture and antibiotic sensitivity. A thorough lavage is then performed; a high flow aspirator/irrigator can loosen purulent adhesions and collect all floating debris. The view afforded by laparoscopy ensures that the entire peritoneal cavity is free of contamination.

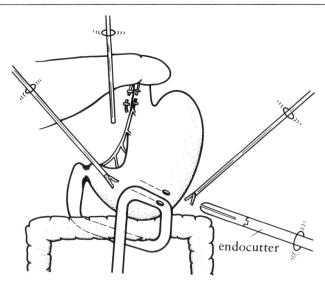

Figure 14.9: Laparoscopic gastroenterostomy: the edges of the gastrostomy and enterostomy are then approximated, after which the defect can be closed and cut clean again with the Endocutter CLC 60.

The perforation is then closed and plugged using two or three sutures. A ski needle with a monofilament absorbable thread is used to take wide bites through the ulcer. The knots are tied intracorporeally over an omental plug (*see* Figure 14.10). Drainage is usually unnecessary. The decision to proceed with a combined anti-ulcer operation depends upon three factors – age, associated medical diseases and time delay since perforation[15].

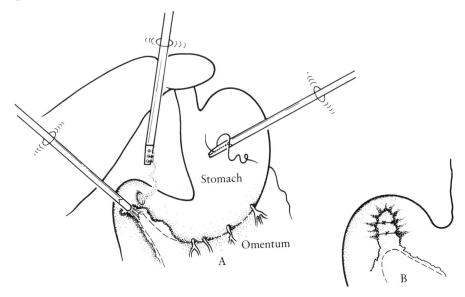

Figure 14.10: In the management of perforated duodenal ulcer: (A) the perforation is closed and plugged using two or three sutures. A ski needle with a monofilament absorbable thread is used to take wide bits through the ulcer. (B) The knots are tied intracorporeally over an omental plug.

Elderly patients with cardiovascular or pulmonary disease, and who present after a delay of 12 hours, are regarded as at high risk, and receive a simple patching of the perforation. Other patients regarded as at low risk receive an anti-ulcer operation as long as the peritoneal contaminant is not purulent.

Postoperative care

The nasogastric tube is left *in situ* for an average of 24 hours following vagotomy alone and 48 hours after closure of an acute duodenal perforation. The patient is discharged two or three days after vagotomy and five days after closure of perforation. Postoperative pain is minimal with the injection of local anaesthetic into the puncture sites.

Repeat endoscopy is performed four to six weeks postoperatively to confirm healing of the ulcer. Postoperative secretory studies are also performed to document reduction in acid output.

Results

By February 1993, we had performed 103 operations for duodenal ulcer at Hospital St Roch. Of these procedures, 78 were performed in patients with chronic duodenal ulcer disease intractable to medical treatment and 28 were performed for acute perforations. All endoscopic evidence of duodenal ulcer was found to have disappeared. One month after the laparoscopic procedure, acid secretion studies – performed in all patients – found a reduction of acid secretion by an average of 80%. No mortality or serious morbidity was observed. Minor complications included pneumothorax, mild diarrhoea (in three patients) and food bezoars requiring endoscopic treatment (in three patients). One patient required surgery for gastro-oesophageal reflux two months postvagotomy. In 19 patients available for long-term follow-up (average two years), one recurrent ulcer has been identified.

Conclusion

We consider that laparoscopic treatment offers patients an excellent chance of controlling their ulcer disease with minimal disruption of their lifestyle. The procedure is quick and reliable, it is performed with basic laparoscopic equipment, and it should be widely effective in the general surgical community. Our current results with the technique show ulcer healing was achieved in all patients. However, data concerning the long-term risks of developing recurrent ulceration, and the results of prospective randomized trials comparing medical and surgical therapy, are keenly awaited.

References

1   Katkhouda N and Mouiel J (1991) Laparoscopic truncal and selective vagotomy. In: Zucker KA, Bailey RW and Reddick EJ, eds. *Surgical laparoscopy*. Quality Medical Publishing, St Louis.

2   Price C and Elder JB (1991) Effect of cimetidine on peptic ulcer surgery in the North-West of England. *Gut.* **22**:A879.

3   Valerio D, Mendry WS and Kyle J (1982) Gastroduodenal perforation in North-East Scotland, 1972–81: a rise in incidence. *Gut.* **23**:A438–A439.

4   Katkhouda N and Mouiel J (1991) Treatment of chronic duodenal ulcer with posterior truncal vagotomy and anterior seromyotomy without laparotomy using video coelioscopy. *Ann. J. Surg.* **161**:361–4.

5   Taylor TV, Lythgoe JP, MC Farrard JB, Gilmore IT, Thouas PE and Ferguson GH (1990) Anterior lesser curve seromyotomy and posterior truncal vagotomy versus truncal vagotomy and pyloroplasty in the treatment of chronic duodenal ulcer disease. *Br. J. Surg.* **77**:1007–9.

6   Gunn AA and Siriwardema AK (1988) Anterior lesser curve seromyotomy and posterior truncal vagotomy for chronic duodenal ulcer: the results at five years. *Br. J. Surg.* **75**:866–8.

7   Oostvogel HJM, Vam Vroomhovem TJMU (1988) Anterior lesser curve seromyotomy with posterior truncal vagotomy versus proximal gastric vagotomy. *Br. J. Surg.* **75**:121–4.

8   Bailey RW, Flowers JL and Graham SM (1991) Combined laparoscopic cholecystectomy and selective vagotomy. *Surg. Laparosc. Endosc.* **1**:45–9.

9   Hill GL and Barker CJ (1978) Anterior highly selective vagotomy with posterior truncal vagotomy: a simple technique for denervating the parietal cell mass. *Br. J. Surg.* **65**:702–5.

10 Taylor TV, Gunn AA and Macleed DAD (1982) Anterior lesser curve seromyotomy and posterior truncal vagotomy in the treatment of chronic duodenal ulcer. *Lancet* **2**:846–8.

11 Taylor TV, Holt S and Heading RC (1985) Gastric emptying after anterior lesser curve seromyotomy and posterior truncal vagotomy. *Br. J. Surg.* **72**:620–2.

12 Kalwaji F and Grange D (1987) Ulcère duodénal chronique. Traitement par seromyotomie fundique antérieure avec vagotomie tronculaire postérieure. *Press Méd.* **16**:28–30.

13 Taylor TV (1983) Experience with the under quist ownman dilator in the upper gastrointestinal. *Br. J. Surg.* **70**:445.

14 Mouiel J, Katkhouda N, White S and Dumas R (1992) Endolaparoscopic palliation of pancreatic cancer. *Surg. Laparosc. Endosc.* **2**:241–3.

15 Boey J, Wong J and Ong GB (1982) A prospective study of operatic risk factor in perforated duodenal ulcer. *Ann. Surg.* **195**:265–9.

15

Laparoscopic Splenectomy

M. MOUNIR GAZAYERLI, HOSAM S. HELMY, MOHAMED HAKKI, and MARY LOU SPITZ

Introduction

With the recent explosion of interest in laparoscopic surgery, it was inevitable that surgeons around the world would, simultaneously and independently of each other, tackle the spleen laparoscopically. The spleen invites laparoscopic removal because it is essentially intraperitoneal, its hilum is easy to dissect, it lies against the parietal peritoneum (thus allowing lateral traction to expose the hilum), and steps can be taken to ensure that it is removed safely.

Indications for splenectomy

Splenectomy is indicated[1,2,3] if there is excessive splenic destruction of blood cells or massive splenomegaly (ie symptomatic splenomegaly or hypersplenism), and also in cases of splenic tumours and abscesses, ruptures and hereditary spherocytosis. It should also be considered in cases of congenital or acquired haemolytic anaemias, acquired thrombocytopenia, primary or secondary hypersplenism, and splenic cysts. It is *not* indicated[2] in cases of glucose-6-phosphate dehydrogenase deficiency, portal hypertension, thalassaemia minor, or chronic myelogenous or granulocytic leukaemia.

Congenital haemolytic anaemias

Hereditary spherocytosis, elliptocytosis (ovalocytosis) and hereditary stomato-cytosis[2-7] are due to red blood cell (RBC) membrane defects. These are autosomal dominant traits. Other anaemias are due to enzyme defects (as in the case of pyruvate kinase deficiency) and abnormal haemoglobins (eg sickle cell anaemia and thalassaemia major or Cooley's anaemia).

In sickle cell anaemia[2,3,5,7], normal HbA is replaced by HbS and, with decreased oxygen tension, HbS undergoes crystallization. Repeated stasis causes splenic infarction (autosplenectomy), and operative splenectomy should generally be avoided in children under five years old. Splenectomy is indicated only in cases of sequestration crisis in infants and small children. In thalassaemia major[3], severe haemolytic anaemia is caused by the persistence of HbF and the reduction of HbA levels. Because of the high incidence of cholelithiasis, concomitant cholecystectomy may be required, so it is important to have an ultrasound done preoperatively.

Acquired haemolytic anaemias

This may consist of Evan's syndrome[2] (a combination of haemolytic anaemia and thrombocytopenia or neutropenia), or idiopathic autoimmune condition resulting from decreased RBC survival because of antibody and/or complement binding to the RBC membrane.

Acquired thrombocytopenia

In idiopathic thrombocytopenic purpura (ITP)[1-5,7-9], antiplatelet IgG produced by the spleen results in splenic sequestration and the destruction of platelets. Acute cases are characterized by a sudden and rapid onset in children aged between two and five years, which remits within six months in 90 % of cases. Intravenous gamma globulin is the treatment of choice; plasma exchange is more effective than in chronic cases, but steroids may not always be effective. Unlike the chronic form, steroids are ineffective. Emergency splenectomy is indicated where the haemorrhage is life-threatening.

Chronic ITP is the most common cause of isolated thrombocytopenia, and spontaneous remission is rare. It is two or three times more common in women than in men, and is most common between 20 and 40 years of age. It should be treated first by steroids, to raise the platelet count and to induce remission of bleeding. If steroids do not work, if there is a relapse or if high doses are required to maintain the platelet count, then splenectomy should be performed. Even after splenectomy, however, there is a 10 % chance of relapse which may be due to accessory spleens, present in 30 % of cases, and they should be searched for during surgery. Immunosuppressive agents are the third line of treatment, either if splenectomy fails or if it is contraindicated. Vincristine is most effective, but other useful drugs are azathioprine, cyclosphamide and danazol.

Patients with AIDS present with classic ITP, but fewer than 10 % of cases respond to steroids[2,3,9] and splenectomy is therefore indicated.

Thrombotic thrombocytopenic purpura (TTP)[1,2,3,5,8] due to subendothelial hyalinization of arterioles with platelet trapping results in arteriole occlusion and thrombocytopaenia. It is characterized by the classic pentad of fever, TTP, haemolytic anaemia, neurological disturbance and renal failure. If it does not respond to plasmapheresis with fresh frozen plasma to remove the causative platelet aggregating factor von Willebrand's factor, steroids and Dextran 70 may be effective.

Hypersplenism

In primary hypersplenism[1–5], which is a diagnosis of exclusion, enlargement of the spleen is associated with deficiency of one or more blood cell types due to splenic sequestration. Secondary hypersplenism[1,5,10], due to a specific disease process, is more complex. It results in hypermetabolism, increased cardiac output, decreased renal perfusion, portal hypertension and dilutational anaemia.

Splenectomy is indicated where there are the following:

1   anaemia, thrombocytopenia, granulocytopaenia
2   hypermetabolism, high-output cardiac decompensation
3   mechanical compression of the stomach, with recurrent painful splenic infarcts
4   bleeding oesophageal or gastric varices.

Causes of secondary hypersplenism are multiple. Splenic vein thrombosis[1,3,5] is most commonly due to pancreatitis, and may present with bleeding oesophageal varices. Neoplastic causes[3,5,6,11] include hairy cell leukaemia; chronic lymphocytic leukaemia; non-Hodgkin's lymphoma, where the neoplasm is composed of monoclonal B-cells classified as nodular (favourable) and diffuse (unfavourable); and agnogenic myeloid metaplasia, which is a myeloproliferative disorder causing progressive fibrosis and sclerosis of the marrow, resulting in extramedullary haemotopoiesis which induces splenomegaly.

HODGKIN'S LYMPHOMA

According to Rye's hystopathologic classification[1], the best prognosis is in cases where the lymphocytes are predominant; the worst, where lymphocytes are depleted. Between thes two extremes, the lymphoma may be nodular sclerosing or of mixed cellularity.

The Ann Arbor staging classification[1,3,5,7] categorizes the lymphoma according to the site and number of lymph node (LN) regions as well as the presence or absence of systemic symptoms.

Stage I: one or two LN regions.
Stage II: more than two LN regions on the same side of the diaphragm.
Stage III: LNs on both sides of the diaphragm, or spleen involvement.
Stage IV: extranodal sites (eg liver or bone marrow).

At the classic staging laparotomy[3,7], the surgeon performs splenectomy with a 2 cm wedge biopsy of the left lobe of the liver and a Tru-Cut needle biopsy of both lobes. Lymph-node sampling is done at the splenic and liver hila, including the cystic duct and the common bile duct LNs; as well as along the coeliac axis and the paraortic, mesenteric, mesocolic and iliac LNs. The procedure concludes with an iliac crest biopsy. Oophoropexy is indicated in premenopausal women, to avoid the risk of sterility during postoperative radiation treatment.

MISCELLANEOUS DISEASES

Felty's syndrome[1,3,5,7] consists of a triad of rheumatoid arthritis, spleno-megaly and neutropenia. Splenectomy is indicated if there are serious or refractory infections, regardless of neutrophil count, or intractable leg ulcers, or where haemolytic anaemia is refractory to transfusions.

Infiltrative diseases[1,3,11] inducing hypersplenism are amyloidosis, sarcoid-osis, and Gaucher's disease (abnormal retention of glycolipid cerebrosides in reticulo-endothelial cells). There is also the congenital disorder erythropoietic porphyria, where RBC pyrole metabolism causes premature RBC destruction in the spleen resulting in haemolysis and splenomegaly.

Splenic cysts

Splenic cysts[5,6,11] larger than 10 cm have a high risk of rupturing. Pseudocysts, due to prior injury, account for 50 to 75 % of cases. True cysts are either parasitic (most often echinococcal) or nonparasitic (eg epidermoid cysts).

Operative technique

Special instrumentation

The operating theatre should be equipped with an extracorporeal knot-ting device (*see* Figure 15.5) and a linear vascular stapling device. A 45° laparoscope, although not essential, greatly facilitates the procedure. The surgeon (and patient) will also be helped greatly if there is a radiology department capable of selective embolization of the splenic artery.

Port placement

If only a splenectomy is contemplated, four or five ports are used: these typically include three 10 or 10–11 mm ports and one 12 or 11–12 mm port. They should ideally form an arc, with the splenic hilum at the centre. Flexibility is essential, however, so the site of the three 10 mm ports will depend on the body habitus. If the xiphoid and the umbilicus are far enough apart for a port to be placed between them without hampering instrument movement, one port should be just below the xiphoid, another at the umbilical scar and the third half-way between them to the right of the rectus muscle (*see* Figure 15.1). Alternatively, one port may be just below the xiphoid, one directly above the umbilicus and to the left of the rectus muscle. The 12 mm port, in the left anterior axillary line, completes the arc; it is used for lateral traction on the spleen during hilar dissection, and the linear stapler is passed through it to transect the hilar vessels. A fifth port (often a 5 mm one) may be placed at the costal margin to aid in the dissection.

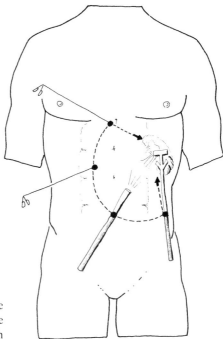

Figure 15.1: Ports in an arc, with the splenic hilum at the centre. There should be at least a hand's width between each port.

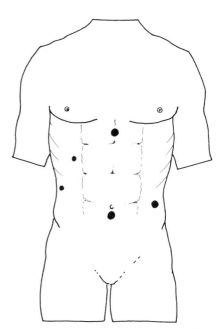

Figure 15.2: If cholecystectomy is performed concomitantly, the surgeon should try to use the midclavicular port for his right hand, although today's instruments may be too short (at 33 cm). A 12 mm anterior axillary port is inserted on completion of the cholecystectomy.

If a cholecystectomy is also to be done, this is carried out first. Here the epigastric and umbilical ports should be in the operating arc, while the midclavicular port can be used for posterior traction on the hilar structures or for the inferomedial traction on the greater curvature of the stomach. The 12 mm anterior axillary port is inserted after the cholecystectomy has been completed (*see* Figure 15.2).

Port assignment

The surgeon usually stands to the right of the patient and uses the high and low midline ports for his left and right hands respectively. The 45° laparoscope is introduced through the left pararectal port. The assistant, who stands to the patient's left side with the camera operator, manipulates the instruments through the 12 mm left anterior axillary port and the optional subcostal port. If extra traction is needed (eg in obese patients), a right pararectal midepigastric trocar can be handled by the camera operator.

However, while these assignments have proved to be effective and comfortable, often the port usage will need to be changed during a procedure. Flexibility is essential to respond to exposure needs and anatomical variations.

Surgical anatomy

The spleen lies along the long axis of the left ninth rib close to the diaphragm. The pathological spleen varies considerably in size: it may be as small as the palm of the hand, or completely fill the abdomen from the left upper quadrant to the right lower quadrant. In a moderately enlarged spleen, the hilar vessels curve forwards: but the possible advantages of this are far outweighed by the difficulty of bagging the enlarged spleen. Extreme enlargement of the spleen, in fact, is a relative contraindication to laparoscopic splenectomy.

If one imagines the spine of a binder or book, the spleen can be compared to an outgrowth from it, with the front cover of the book being the gastrosplenic ligament containing the short gastric vessels, and the back cover being the lienorenal ligament containing the splenic artery and vein. The upper pole of the spleen is attached to the diaphragm by the lienophrenic ligament, while the lower pole is attached to the colon by the lienocolic ligament. These two ligaments have no named vessels and they are usually relatively avascular, although they can be very vascular in cases of hypersplenism. One potential problem comes from the adhesions which may develop between the diaphragm and the lateral surface of the spleen. The phrenicocolic ligament is not attached to the spleen, but cradles its lower pole, forming the boundary of the splenic fossa (*see* Figure 15.3).

Dissection

First an abdominal exploration is carried out to inspect the contents and to look for accessory spleens that might or might not have shown up on the preoperative CT scan. If no preoperative embolization of the splenic artery has been done, the first step should be to enter the lesser sac and clip or ligate the splenic artery in continuity at the upper border of the pancreas. For the inexperienced surgeon, and when dealing with large spleens, it is advisable to embolize the splenic artery and eliminate this step.

The assistant then uses the the left anterior axillary port to retract the spleen laterally to provide countertraction (*see* Figure 15.1). The surgeon dissects the short gastric vessels and individually ligates or clips them, to transsect them (*see* Figure 15.4) and thereby allow exposure of the hilum.

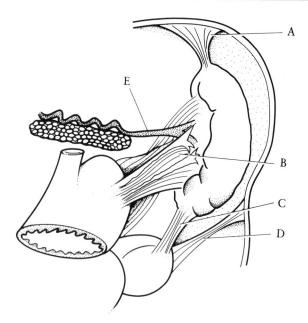

Figure 15.3: A: lienophrenic (splenophrenic) ligament attaches upper pole of spleen to diaphragm. B: lienogastric (gastrosplenic) ligament is the anterior leaf of the splenic hilum and contains the shorter vessels. C: the lienocolic (splencolic) ligament attaches lower pole of spleen to splenic flexure of colon. D: phrenocolic ligament supports lower pole of spleen if the spleen is not too enlarged. It forms the lower boundary of splenic fossa. E: lienorenal (splenorenal) ligament is the posterior leaf of splenic hilum and contains the splenic vessels as they run from the tail of the pancreas to the spleen.

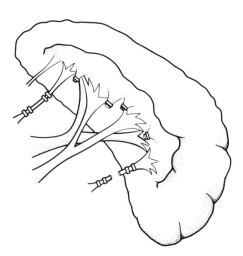

Figure 15.4: Short gastric vessels are divided between clips, exposing splenic artery and vein.

If a preoperative embolization has been carried out, the arteriogram will also indicate the number of splenic vessels and their anatomical pattern. Once the vessels have been dissected they are ligated, preferably using extracorporeal knots (*see* Figure 15.5). The artery and veins can be ligated together if preoperative embolization has been done; otherwise they must

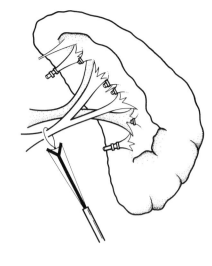

Figure 15.5: Splenic artery is ligated, preferably by an extracorporeal knot pusher (eg the Gazayerli knot pusher, V Mueller Inc, Chicago).

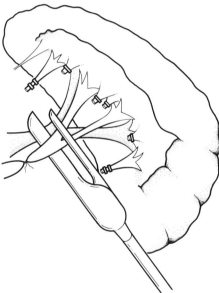

Figure 15.6: Splenic artery is divided by a linear vascular stapler. The splenic vein is similarly ligated and then divided.

be ligated individually to prevent arteriovenous fistula formation. This is followed by stapling and transsection by means of a linear vascular stapling device (*see* Figure 15.6). However, the use of clips alone on the splenic vessels is hazardous as they can be dislodged easily during subsequent manipulation. The different viewing angle provided by a 45° scope allows for excellent visualization of the hilum and the upper and lower poles of the spleen and any attachments to them. Our routine has been first to tackle the short gastric vessels below the hilum, then the hilum itself, and then to mobilize the lower pole of the spleen, followed by the short gastrics above the hilum with the attachments to the upper pole. This leaves relatively avascular posterior attachments that need to be divided to free the spleen completely. One of the most satisfying sights is to see the spleen somersautling freely in its bed. Then comes the task of removing the spleen from the abdominal cavity.

Extraction of the spleen

It is not always easy to place the spleen into a plastic bag to remove it, but we have managed it in all cases operated on to date. When the spleen is small, as in cases of ITP, the spleen is relatively easily placed in the new large Pleatman sac (provided by Cabot), but further improvements are needed. Currently the largest available sac measures 10 × 10 cm. We have asked the manufacturers to provide sacs measuring 15 × 15 cm or even 20 × 20 cm. We are also hoping that they will add a wire mechanism along the opening, to keep the sac open. In hypersplenism and spherocytosis, spleens are larger and pose more of a challenge. Sometimes we have been able to put a suction tip into the spleen, to suck out a large part of the spleen pulp without spillage and then to lift up the flabby splenic capsule and place it in the sac. Once the spleen is in there, the opening of the sac is brought out from a port site (usually the left anterior axillary one), and evacuation of the spleen is carried out by means of suction, finger fracture or instrument fracture, after which extraction is performed with an ovum forceps (see Figure 15.7). If an intact spleen is needed for pathological examination, it can usually be squeezed out of

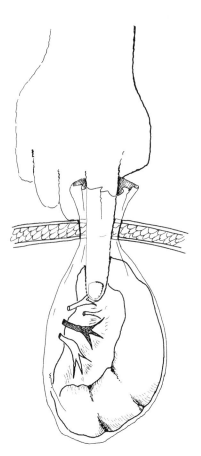

Figure 15.7: Spleen is placed into a plastic bag and either suctioned or broken and extracted. The incision can be enlarged slightly to squeeze and remove an intact spleen for pathological examination if necessary.

an incision no larger than 5 cm. Copious irrigation is performed without drainage.

Results

We have now attempted 14 procedures and completed them all successfully. Embolization of the splenic artery has been carried out in six cases, five with coils and one with a detachable balloon. Six of the cases procedures have been for familial spherocytosis, seven for ITP and one for schistosomiasis with hypersplenism. One of the patients with ITP posed a particular challenge, because she had a total pelvic exenteration with a colostomy and ileal loop diversion. Her presenting platelet count was 26 000 per μl on steroid therapy. In spite of the restricted abdominal cavity, the splenectomy was carried out successfully and she was discharged 36 hours later with a platelet count of 96 000 per μl.

References

1   Carabasi RA III (1991) Spleen. In: Jarell BE, Carabasi RA III, *Surgery*, 2nd edn. Williams & Wilkins, Baltimore. pp.371–7.

2   Graham RA and Hohn DC (1989) Splenectomy for hematologic disorders. In: Cameron JL (ed.) *Current surgical therapy*, 3rd edn. Decker, Philadelphia. pp.399–403.

3   Sheldon GF, Croom RD and Meyer AA (1986) The spleen. In: Sabiston DC (ed.) *Textbook of surgery: the biological basis of modern surgical practice*, 13th edn. WB Saunders, Philadelphia. pp1203–30.

4   Ballinger WF (1992) Splenectomy for hematologic disorders. In: Cameron JL (ed.) *Current surgical therapy*, 4th edn. CV Mosby — Year Book, St Louis. pp.513–17.

5   Meyer AA (1992) Spleen. In: Greenfield LJ *et al.* (eds.) Surgery, scientific principles and practice. JB Lippincott, Philadelphia. pp.1142–61.

6   Raytch RF (1992) Tumors, cysts and abscesses of the spleen. In: Cameron JL (ed.) *Current surgical therapy*, 4th edn. CV Mosby — Year Book, St Louis. pp.518–21.

7   Schwartz SI (1989) *Principles of surgery*, 5th edn. McGraw Hill, New York. pp.1141–57.

8   Bithell TC (1987) Disorders of platelets. In: Thorup OA (ed.) *Leavell and Thorup's fundamentals of clinical hematology*, 5th edn. WB Saunders, Philadelphia. pp.792–806.

9   Shulman NR and Jordan JV (1987) Platelet immunology. In: Coleman RW *et al.* (eds) *Hemostasis and thrombosis: basic principles and clinical practice*, 2nd edn. JB Lippincott, Philadelphia. pp.491–529.

10   Hess CE (1987) Splenomegaly. In: Thorup OA (ed.) *Leavell and Thorup's fundamentals of clinical hematology*, 5th edn. WB Saunders, Philadelphia. pp.557–71.

11   Aldrete JS (1989) Cysts and abscesses of the spleen. In: Cameron JL (ed.) *Current surgical therapy*, 3rd edn. Decker, Philadelphia. pp.403–7.

16

Laparoscopic Adrenalectomy

DAVID R. FLETCHER

Indications for adrenalectomy

The indications for adrenalectomy, and its surgical management, have changed dramatically over recent years as a result of advances in pharmacology and in imaging, and soon they may change even more with the advent of laparoscopic surgery. For example, the development of anti-oestrogens means that the adrenals are no longer removed for palliation of breast cancer. While hyperfunction is still best managed by excision, this management has become easier for the surgeon, due to advances is hormone assay of plasma and urine (to establish the diagnosis) and in imaging (to localize the site of the lesion). This allows the optimal surgical approach to be planned. Conn's tumours, for example, which produce aldosterone, are invariably unilateral, intra-adrenal and usually easily localized on CT scan; while Cushing's syndrome is due to adrenal tumour in only 20 % of cases, the rest being caused by adrenal hyperplasia (due either to ACTH-producing pituitary micro or macro adenomata, or to ectopic ACTH production by para-endocrine tumours)[1]. In these circumstances, bilateral adrenal excision would be required when the site of ACTH production could not be controlled surgically and pharmacologic blockade of adrenal cortisol was no longer appropriate. Medullary tumours (mostly phaeochromocytoma) are more complicated in that they may be extra-adrenal as well as bilateral, particularly in the multiple endocrine neoplasia type II syndrome. The requirement for surgeons to perform extensive abdominal exploration at operation to exclude extra-adrenal tumours[2] has decreased with the advent of MIBG scanning[3].

A second major indication for adrenalectomy is the management of an adrenal mass which is either symptomatic or which has been discovered on CT scan or ultrasound performed for other purposes. The quality of the CT image is now such that adrenal masses are identified in 2 % of all abdominal CT scans[4–6]. Once identified, symptomatic or incidental, there is a need to exclude hyperfunction or malignancy. Lesions smaller than 1 cm are unlikely to be functional, and should not be investigated further hormonally (apart from 24-hour urine VMA and catechols) unless specific clinical symptoms are present[4-6]. Occasionally CT scans may suggest that the lesion is either benign (cyst or adrenolipoma) or malignant (invasion of tissue planes, metastases), but usually they cannot differentiate between benign and malignant disease. Therefore, rather than perform percutaneous CT-guided biopsy which has a substantial false negative rate, all adrenal lesions 6 cm or larger should be removed to exclude malignancy[4-6]. The larger the lesion, the greater the chance of malignancy. Non-functioning adrenal lesions smaller than 6 cm, meanwhile, need to be followed by serial CT scan.

Surgical approaches to the adrenal

Small, benign and accurately localized lesions are best managed by a posterior approach excising the 12th rib[1]. Pain and morbidity are relatively minor and the cosmetic result is reasonable. Cushing's syndrome due to hyperplasia can be managed similarly by a bilateral posterior approach. To ensure adequate exposure and clearance, large tumours – particularly those which are potentially malignant – are best managed by a lateral approach, excising the 11th rib on the left and the 10th rib on the right[1]. Familial bilateral phaeochromocytoma, with extra-adrenal tumour on MIBG or CT scan, are best managed by anterior laparotomy to ensure that all abnormal catechol-producing tissue is excised[1,2].

The role of the laparoscope

The appeal of being able to remove or repair a viscus without creating a large and painful wound to access it has resulted in the rapid development of therapeutic laparoscopic techniques[7,8]. Not all procedures, however, are necessarily appropriate for the laparoscopic approach. Potentially suitable procedures are first those in which the pathology can be safely and effectively managed with laparoscopic instrumentation, and second those in which the major morbidity of the alternative procedure was due to the wound of access. According to these criteria, a laparoscopic approach is suitable for well localized hyperfunctional adrenal tumours and non-functional adrenal lesions or 'incidentalomas' larger than 6 cm. Bilateral lesions can and have been removed laparoscopically[9], which is reasonable so long as extra-adrenal localization has been excluded in cases of phaeochromocytoma. The possible cost of extra operating time has to be balanced against the predicted benefit of earlier discharge from hospital and return to productive activity. However, the removal of possible adrenal carcinomas should not be attempted laparoscopically. It is not worth saving a few days in hospital if this increases the incidence of tumour recurrence, either locally or in a wound. Surgical principles should not be compromised just so that the procedure can be performed laparoscopically. The operation has to be designed to suit the pathology, not vice versa.

Operative technique

Excess hormone production, particularly of catecholamines, must be controlled prior to and during surgery. Prophylactic low-dose heparin should be started before surgery, and calf stimulators used during surgery, because of reports of an increased incidence of deep venous thrombosis and pulmonary embolus associated with prolonged laparoscopic surgery and pneumoperitoneum.

In the first two procedures performed by the author, as recommended by Pételin[10], the patient was placed in the lithotomy position, using the Lloyd-Davies table; the surgeon sat between the legs, and the camera operator and assistant sat on either side. The patient was rotated using a sand bag on the ipsilateral side and then strapped to the operating table. The next two procedures performed by the author used a lateral approach, modified from that described by Gagner[11]. This approach has considerable advantage. First, the mobilized spleen/pancreas on the left or liver on the right do not need to be laboriously elevated on retractors, since gravity assists in their displacement. Second, any blood drains away, keeping the operative field clear, rather than pooling in the dependent adrenal bed. Only the lateral approach, therefore, will be described for each side.

The patient is placed on his or her side on a well padded operating table, the side of the abnormal adrenal uppermost. The front of the patient's chest and abdomen must be at the edge of the operating table, to allow the tips of instruments to be angled upwards without the handles striking the operating table. Calf stimulators are attached to the legs and then a pillow is placed between the legs. The uppermost arm is supported on a thoracic arm-rest and placed above the face out of the operative field. The patient is then strapped to the table. The surgeon stands facing the patient's abdomen. If an assistant is required to retract the spleen or liver, s/he will stand on the same side as the surgeon, opposite the patient's chest. The camera operator and scrub nurse are at the patient's back.

A 10 mm Hasson cannula (positon 1, *see* Figures 16.1, 16.2) is placed in the umbilicus. The alternative is Veress needle insufflation and blind cannulation in the upper quadrant, though this may increase the chance of intestinal injury. A cannula placed at the umbilicus also has the advantage of allowing extension of the incision if necessary to remove a big lesion without significant cosmetic disturbance. Finally, it allows accurate placement of subsequent cannulae. By placing an infiltration needle through the abdominal wall under vision, the ideal distance from and angle to the adrenal for instruments can be selected. The chosen area can then be infiltrated with local anaesthetic to decrease postoperative pain further. Four more cannulae are inserted as indicated in Figures 16.1 and 16.2. On the left side, they will need to be placed further from the costal margin.

After placement of the Hasson cannula, for left adrenalectomy cannulae 3 and

4 are inserted (*see* Figures 16.1). Note that cannula 4 is approximately in the mid-axillary line. This cannula will be used for scissors, CUSA (Cavitron Ultrasonic Surgical Aspirator, Valley Lab., Australia) and clip applier. Cannula 3 will be used for a dissector and suction irrigator. Using scissors and a dissector in cannulae 3 and 4 (*see* Figure 16.1), any adhesions between spleen and diaphragm are now taken down and the splenic flexure and descending colon are mobilized, allowing the colon to drop toward the midline exposing the paracolic gutter. With the colon mobilized, a 10 mm cannula is placed well lateral and posterior in position 5 (*see* Figure 16.1). It can now be used for the laparoscope. The advantage of this position is that it places the camera operator out of the surgeon's field of activity and gives a superb direct view of the adrenal, close to the line of the surgeon's instruments in cannulae 3 and 4 (*see* Figure 16.1).

The assistant passes a Du Val bowel grasper through cannula 1 in the umbilicus, grasps the splenic flexure and displaces the colon inferiorly. The surgeon then mobilizes the lienorenal ligament using scissors in cannula 4 and a dissector in cannula 3. The effect of gravity is to allow the spleen to drop towards the midline, exposing the tail of the pancreas, which is very easily seen

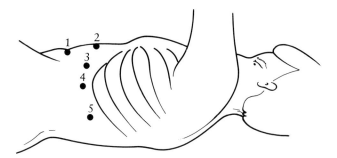

Figure 16.1: Placement of 10 mm cannulae for performance of left adrenalectomy. The surgeon faces the patient and works through cannuale 3 and 4. The camera operator stands behind the patient with the scrub nurse, with the camera placed in cannula 5. Retraction of spleen and pancreas or adrenal is via cannula 1 or optionally cannula 2.

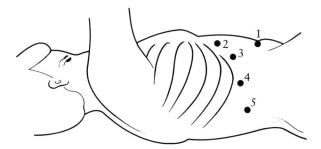

Figure 16.2: Placement of 10 mm cannulae for performance of right adrenalectomy. The surgeon faces the patient working through cannulae 3 and 4. The camera operator stands behind the patient with the scrub nurse, with the camera placed in cannula 5. Retraction of liver or adrenal is via cannula 1 or optionally cannula 2. Note that the cannulae are closer to the costal margin than on the left side.

with the laparoscope in cannula 5. If this does not happen, despite adequate mobilization, another 10 mm cannula will need to be placed in position 2 (*see* Figure 16.1) for a fan retractor. The space between the tail of the pancreas and kidney is next gently deepened using the scissors and dissector in cannulae 3 and 4. This may require mobilization of the terminal part of the transverse colon. This tissue frequently contains vessels to the lower pole of the spleen and usually requires the application of clips before division. The plane anterior to the kidney is deepened superiorly toward the upper pole of the kidney. The typical brown adrenal tissue will usually pop into view when the perirenal tissue is opened. This fatty tissue (excessive in the obese) should be mobilized from the adrenal.

If a normal piece of adrenal presents itself first, it may be gently grasped in a broad grasper (eg Du Val) passed via cannula 1 in the umbilicus (if it will reach) or via the optional cannula 2 (*see* Figure 16.1). In the latter situation, if retraction is required, the retractor may be passed via cannula 1 in the umbilicus and held by the scrub nurse or second assistant whilst the camera operator holds the adrenal with the Du Val in cannula 2 (*see* Figure 16.1). The main adrenal vein passing to the left renal vein is then identified using a right-angle dissector passed via cannula 4 to tease away fat and tissue along the inferior edge of the adrenal. It is wise to clip this main vein early, as handling the adrenal – even in non-catechol producing tumours – can produce marked changes in blood pressure (one of the author's patients with a Cushing's tumour had systolic blood pressure rises of 60 mmHg). If the tumour presents itself first, however, it is unwise to grasp it with a dissector or grasper as the tumour easily fragments and leads to bleeding. Not only may this obscure the view: more importantly it may seed tumour fragments, resulting in syndrome recurrence. When the adrenal cannot be grasped, it is preferable to displace the tumour superiorly away from the renal vein using a sucker passed via cannula 1 or 2. The CUSA is ideal for dissecting the vessels. Its tip oscillates at 25 000 cycles per second, which fragments tissue with a high water content and leaves the fibrous tissue of blood vessels intact. Fat and fluid are aspirated, exposing the vessels to be mobilized. The CUSA is removed from cannula 4 and a clip applier is inserted, to place two clips across the vessel which is then divided with scissors. Small vessels can be controlled with diathermy either via the dissecting forceps in cannula 3 or via the CUSA itself.

Once the inferior edge has been freed, anterior and posterior planes are created using an instrument in cannula 3 to displace the gland and the CUSA or dissector in cannula 4. On the medial side, further vessels may need to be clipped and divided passing directly to the aorta.

Once the gland has been freed, a bag is passed into the abdomen via cannula 1 at the umbilicus. Using a grasper in cannula 3 (and 2 if present), the bag is held open whilst the grasper in cannula 4 places the specimen in the bag. The bed of the adrenal is then lavaged, and all fluid and blood removed, following which the specimen is removed under vision. A larger tumour may require extension of the umbilical incision as well as fragmentation of the tumour within the bag once the neck of that bag has been delivered through the umbilicus. Ideally this is done with instruments such as a sponge holder which is then not used again, so as to avoid possible tumour seeding. It is also done under view with the laparoscope from below, to ensure that the bag is not torn. The umbilical incision is then sutured and the skin closed, and the remaining cannulae removed under vision to make sure that there is no bleeding from them. The cannula sites are then sutured and the skin closed.

The approach is similar on the right side. Following the insertion of the 10 mm Hasson cannula in the umbilicus, cannulae 3 and 4 are inserted (*see* Figure 16.2). On the right side, because of the more cephalad position of the adrenal, these cannulae will be closer to the costal margin than on the left (*see* figure 16.1). The right colon is mobilized if necessary to allow the placement well lateral of the 10 mm cannula at position 5 (*see* Figure 16.2). The laparoscope is then transferred from cannula 1 to cannula 5 and, using scissors in cannula 3 and graspers in cannula 4, the surgeon mobilizes the liver by dividing the triangular ligament (*see* Figure 16.2). Once mobilized, the liver drops towards the midline but may need gentle anterior displacement using a retractor in cannula 2. A Du Val grasper is passed via cannula 1 to pull the hepatic flexure of the colon inferiorly so that the duodenum can be mobilized. This mobilization of the duodenum proceeds until the vena cava comes into view. The cephalad extension of the peritoneum along the edge of the vena cava posterior to the liver is then divided. This should be done cautiously, lifting the peritoneum with the left hand with a dissector in cannula 4 and using the scissors in cannula 3 to dissect under the peritoneum before dividing it. The fat above the kidney rapidly comes into view. The incision in the peritoneum is then extended laterally at the level of the upper pole of the kidney so that the peritoneal flap can be lifted and displaced toward the head. The short right adrenal vein passing to the vena cava should next be identified. This is very easily achieved with the CUSA, which rapidly disposes of the fat; but if it is unavailable, the dissection can proceed with a sucker and a dissector or a dissector and scissors in cannulae 4 and 3 respectively (*see* Figure 16.2). However, all tissue must be lifted and examined before cutting to avoid inadvertent injury to the short adrenal vein. Once the vein has been identified, sufficient length is mobilized using a right-angle dissector in cannula 3 whilst the adrenal is distracted away from the vena cava using a dissector in cannula 4. The vein is double-clipped and divided with scissors. The plane along the edge of the vena cava is then deepened displacing the adrenal away from the cava. Once more, if normal adrenal can be seen, it can be grasped gently with a grasper in cannula 4 (or 2 if present). If only tumour is seen, however, it is best displaced using a sucker so as to avoid fragmentation.

Once the medial plane adjacent to the vena cava has been completed, a caudad plane along the upper pole of the kidney and renal vessels is created. Small branches passing to and from the renal vessels require either clipping or diathermy and then division. Once the caudad and medial planes have been created, the adrenal can be lifted upwards and a posterior plane obtained. Blunt or CUSA dissection rapidly completes this part of the dissection, leaving only the upper pole to be cleared.

Similarly, the specimen is removed via a bag placed via cannula 1 in the umbilicus. Specimen removal, lavage of the bed and removal of cannulae and closure of wounds are performed as on the left side.

Postoperative care and outcome

Hormonal replacement is necessary for patients having bilateral adrenalectomy and those with Cushing's syndrome (in the latter, the dose should be rapidly tapered off). Narcotics are rarely required beyond the first 24 hours, and patients are encouraged to walk early to reduce the risk of deep venous thrombosis. Diet is resumed at will, usually on the first postoperative day, although one patient of the four treated by the author did not eat until the third postoperative day.

From September 1992 to May 1993, five patients were evaluated for laparoscopic adrenalectomy. One patient with a 15 cm left adrenal lesion diagnosed as a result of loin pain had a left 11th rib excision by open operation because the CT scan was suggestive of invasion and therefore malignancy. Four other patients had a laparoscopic resection. Three left adrenals were removed: a 2 cm Conn's tumour in a 47-year-old hypertensive male, a 1.5 cm Cushing's tumour in a 37-year-old female, and a 3 cm Conn's tumour in a 52-year-old hypertensive female; and, on the right side, a 6 cm non-functional, tumour (benign on histology) in a 50-year-old grossly obese, cigarette-smoking, respiratory compromised male.

The first laparoscopic case took 6 1/4 hours, using the supine position. Cases 3 and 4, using a lateral approach, were completed in 4 and 3 hours respectively. Operating times can be expected to get shorter with experience. Blood loss was not measurable in any of the cases.

Three patients (including the heavy smoker) were discharged on day 3, while the Cushing's patient was discharged on day 4. They all returned to normal activity after seven to 10 days. One Conn's patient redeveloped hypertension (150/95) four months postoperatively. This was confirmed to be essential in nature, as evidenced by normal plasma renin activity and aldosterone.

Conclusion

Laparoscopic adrenalectomy is a good example of appropriate minimal access surgery. Early experience suggests that it has the advantages of other established laparoscopic procedures such as cholecystectomy, in that it allows an early discharge from hospital and an early return to normal activity. Like cholecystectomy, however – and despite the minimal access approach and its low morbidity – the procedure performed internally is the same as that performed at open surgery. The potential for injury is therefore the same and, as with cholecystectomy, may even be greater during the introduction of the technique. It is therefore important that indications for surgery are not liberalized as regards the incidentally discovered adrenal lesion. Once an adrenal mass is inadvertently diagnosed, one should resist the 'cascade effect'[4] – the urge to go on and remove everything laparoscopically. Appropriately applied, however, the laparoscope is likely to be yet another major advance in the management of adrenal pathology.

Acknowledgements

The author thanks Gayle Henry for preparation of the manuscript and David Slattery for preparation of the artwork.

References

1   Welbourn RB (1980) Some aspects of adrenal surgery. *Br. J. Surg.* **67**:723–7.

2   Fletcher DR, Gamvros O, Macfarlane A, Ward-McQuaid JN and Lynn J (1984) Results of a screening program for multiple endocrine neoplasm type II. *Surg. Gyn. Obst.* **159**:119–26.

3   Thompson NW, Allo MD, Shapiro B, Sisson JC *et al.* (1984) Extra-adrenal and metastatic pheochromocytoma: the role of ^{131}I meta-iodobenzylguanidine (^{131}I MIBG) in localization and management. *World J. Surg.* **8**:605–11.

4   Ross NS and Aron DC (1990) Hormonal evaluation of the patient with an incidentally discovered adrenal mass. *N. Engl. J. Med.* **323**:1401–5.

5   Gajraj H and Young AE (1993) Adrenal incidentaloma. *Br. J. Surg.* **80**:422–6.

6   Herrera MF, Grant DS, van Heerden JA *et al.* (1991) Incidentally discovered adrenal tumors: an institutional perspective. *Surg.* **110**:1014–21.

7   Katkhouda N, Fabiani P, Benziri E and Mouiel J (1992) Laser resection of a liver hydatid cyst under video laparoscopy. *Br. J. Surg.* **79**:560–1.

8   Fletcher DR and Jones RM (1992) Laparoscopic cholecystjejunostomy as palliation for obstructive jaundice in inoperable carcinoma of pancreas. *Surg. Endosc.* **6**:147–9.

9   Gagner M, Lacroix A and Bolte E (1992) Laparoscopic adrenalectomy in Cushing's syndrome and pheochromocytoma. *N. Engl. J. Med.* **327**:1033. (Letter.)

10 Petelin JB (1992) Laparoscopic adrenalectomy. *Proceedings of the Third World Congress Endoscopic Surgery*, Bordeaux, June. (Abstract 879.)

11 Gagner M (1993) *Proceedings of the Annual Scientific Meeting of the Society of American Gastroendoscopic Surgeons*, Phoenix, Arizona, April.

17

Video-Enhanced Telescopic Surgical Training

DAVID ROSIN

The introduction of laparoscopic cholecystectomy was an important mile-stone in surgical practice and heralded the development of further minimal access techniques. The advantage of this approach in general surgery is the reduction in the trauma of access without compromising the view of the operative field[1]. This means accelerated patient recovery and a reduction in wound-related complications.

Cholecystectomy is the most common elective abdominal operation in England and Wales, with over 50 000 performed each year[2]. In the USA, it is estimated that over 400 000 cholecystectomies are performed annually. It is traditionally the operation in which surgeons in training gain operative experience and confidence. This is also true of hernia repair operations. Over 90 000 hernia repairs are performed annually in England and Wales – an incidence of 100 per 100 000 operations each year. In the USA, this incidence is 280 per 100 000 annually. The most common emergency general surgical operation performed, usually by first-year residents, is appendicectomy. As these operations are now being performed laparoscopically by more senior surgeons, the introduction of laparoscopic surgery into routine practice is having profound effects on surgical training. Over the last few years, senior surgeons have been learning how to perform laparoscopic cholecystectomy, markedly reducing the number of open cholecystectomies available for junior surgeons in training. Conversely, in a few hospitals where laparoscopic cholecystectomy is not practised, surgeons in training are not being exposed to the new laparoscopic surgical techniques which they need to learn and perform.

In December 1990, the Royal College of Surgeons of England published a report welcoming the development of minimal access surgery[3]. They recommended guidelines for training in, and provision of, laparoscopic surgery. These included gaining experience in laparoscopy through attending gynaecological laparoscopy lists, and the acquisition of basic laparoscopic operative skills (by bench trainers) in a skills laboratory. However, this is not necessarily what surgeons in training actually want.

It was felt that before a training programme could be set out, the views and opinions of surgeons in training should be analysed. A questionnaire was structured seeking opinions from junior surgeons regarding training requirements and accreditation necessity, together with their concerns and perceived advantages of laparoscopic surgery. The draft questionnaire was sent to 64 general surgeons in training in the North West Thames Region of England for each training grade (senior registrar, registrar, senior house officer and pre-registration house surgeon). Subsequently, the questionnaire was enlarged to encompass other laparoscopic general surgical procedures and sent to 100 surgeons in training from all parts of England and Wales.

Results of the first questionnaire

To assure a 100% response rate, individuals were contacted directly by telephone after they had received the questionnaire. Twenty-eight surgeons (44%) were working in hospitals where laparoscopic cholecystectomies were performed, with almost equal numbers from each training grade. Three (5%) had performed laparoscopic cholecystectomies and 19 (30%) had assisted at these operations.

Fifty-nine (92%) surgeons in training said that special training in laparoscopy was required prior to performing laparoscopic cholecystectomy. All said that this should be provided by general surgical consultants (*see* Table 17.2). Twenty-one said this should be supplemented by a comprehensive course, but only 20% wanted gynaecologists to train them (*see* Table 17.2). A summary of the results is shown in Tables 17.1–17.5.

---

1. Have you seen, assisted at or performed laparoscopic cholecystectomy?
2. Is special training required for laparoscopic surgery? If so, what?
3. Should laser/diathermy be used? Is special training required for laser surgery? If so, what?
4. Should surgeons be accredited for laparoscopic surgery?
5. What are the advantages of laparoscopic surgery?
6. Do you have any concerns about laparoscopic surgery?

Table 17.1: Survey of surgeons in training: general questions.

	Training by general surgical consultants	Training by gynaecologists	Training as part of a laparo-scopic chole-cystectomy course
Senior registrars	13	0	9
Registrars	15	4	4
SHOs	15	3	3
Pre-registration HSs	6	5	5
Total	59(100%)	12(20%)	21(36%)

Table 17.2: Survey of surgeons in training: 'What should training for laparoscopy consist of?'

	No	Yes	By RCS	By consultant
Senior registrars	15(94%)	1(6%)	0	1
Registrars	10(62%)	6(38%)	2	4
SHOs	4(25%)	12(75%)	9	3
Pre-registration HSs	3(19%)	13(81%)	9	4
Total	32(50%)	32(50%)	20(63%)	12(37%)

Table 17.3: Survey of surgeons in training: 'Should there be accreditation for laparoscopic surgery? If so, who should give it?'

	Reduced hospital stay	Better patient comfort	Quicker return to work	Better cosmetic result	Don't know
Senior registrars	7	7	2	2	2
Registrars	8	2	4	0	3
SHOs	11	2	2	1	5
Pre-registration HSs	10	1	3	1	5
Total	36(56%)	12(19%)	9(14%)	4(6%)	13(20%)

Table 17.4: Survey of surgeons in training: 'What are the advantages of laparoscopic surgery?'

	Being performed by inexperienced consultants	Detrimental effect on juniors' training	Procedures not yet evaluated	None
Senior registrars	10	5	3	0
Registrars	7	3	0	7
SHOs	4	3	0	9
Pre-registration HSs	9	2	1	4
Total	30(47%)	13(20%)	4(6%)	20(31%)

Table 17.5: Survey of surgeons in training: 'What are your concerns about laparoscopic surgery?'

Second questionnaire

This questionnaire was based on the first one, which had been sent out in December 1990, but it was enlarged to include questions on other minimal access general surgical operations. It was sent to 100 registrars and senior registrars, specifically to see whether the wider implementation of video-enhanced telescopic surgery had influenced their training, and indeed to find out what training they had received in minimal access surgery. The questionnaire was sent out in early 1992 and the results were collated by May of that year. Some of the senior registrars had become consultants by the time they filled in these questionnaires.

Results

The questionnaire asked the registrars to consider their concerns about minimal access surgery (Table 17.6); whether they had performed laparoscopic appendicectomy (Table 17.7), diagnostic laparoscopy (Table 17.8), operative cholangiography (Table 17.9); whether they had been taught to perform laparoscopic cholangiography (Table 17.10); their thoughts on accreditation (Table 17.11); whether minimal access surgery affects surgeons in training (Table 17.12) and whether they had joined the new Society of Minimally Invasive General Surgeons (Table 17.13).

	Consultant	Senior registrar	Registrar	Total
Had concerns	74	84	95	87
Being performed by inadequately				
trained surgeons	18	35	28	29
Inappropriate application	18	29	44	29
Less conventional operations				
for junior training	18	20	39	23
Lack of audit	0	18	17	14
Risk of CBD injury	12	12	6	10
May miss coexistent carcinoma	12	6	0	6

(Figures refer to percentage of those concerned)
The perceived advantages of minimal access surgery were reduced: hospital stay (65), return to work time (62) and pain (49)
The perceived disadvantages were increased operating time (64), expense (51) and an increased complication rate (41)

Table 17.6: Survey of surgeons in training: 'What are your concerns about minimal access surgery?' (87% had concerns).

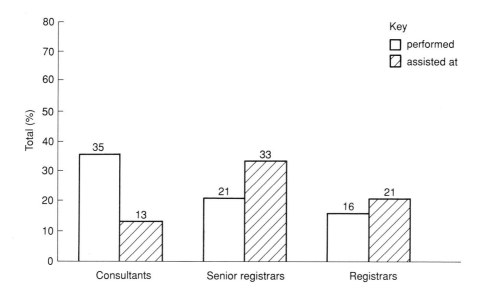

Table 17.7: Survey of surgeons in training: 'Have you performed laparoscopic appendicectomy?'

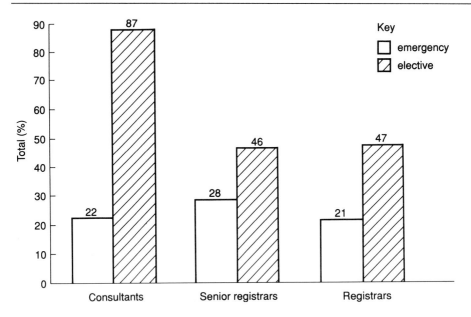

Table 17.8: Survey of surgeons in training: 'Do you perform diagnostic laparoscopy?'

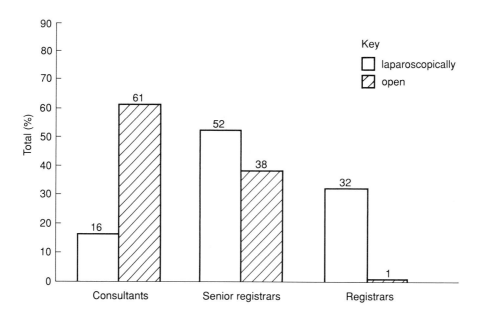

Table 17.9: Survey of surgeons in training: 'Do you perform operative cholangiography?'

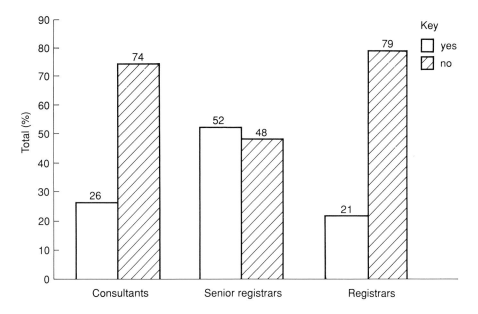

Table 17.10: Survey of surgeons in training: 'Have you been taught laparoscopic cholangiography?'

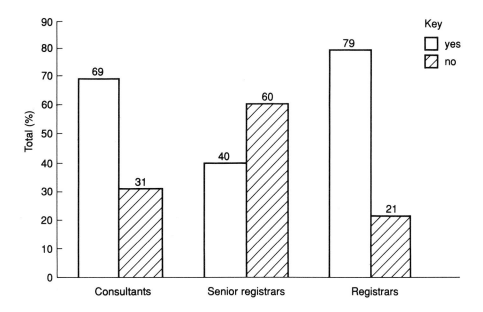

Accreditation should be by: consultant (92%), RCS (60%), an independent course (58%)
10% thought minimal access surgery should be a specialty
A training course was considered necessary by 75%

Table 17.11: Survey of surgeons in training: 'Is accreditation necessary?'

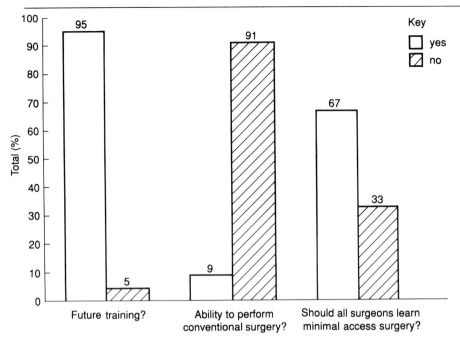

Table 17.12: Survey of surgeons in training: 'Will minimal access surgery affect surgeons' training?'

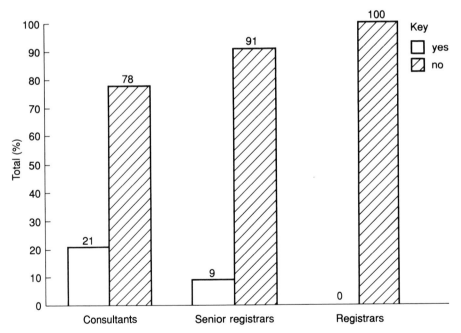

Table 17.13: Survey of surgeons in training: 'Are you a member of the Society of Minimally Invasive General Surgeons?'

87% of respondents had concerns about minimal access surgery, although some of them had not performed any laparoscopic appendicectomies or diagnostic laparoscopies (*see* Table 17.6). It was interesting how few of them had been taught laparoscopic cholangiography and their use of this technique was less than that of routine cholecystectomy.

Those surgeons in training who were still senior registrars, did not believe that accreditation was necessary. All the others did however, and thought it should be given by the consultant in charge.

Most (95%) believed that minimal access surgery would affect their future training but would not affect their ability to perform conventional surgery. 67% felt that all surgeons should learn minimal access techniques.

Few of the 100 surgeons in training had joined the Society of Minimally Invasive General Surgeons (less than a third).

During the last few years, laparoscopic general surgery has gained rapid acceptance and is being performed widely by general surgeons, even in the UK where traditions are slow to change. No advance in recent memory has engendered such widespread interest and debate as has laparoscopic cholecystectomy.

The first time a large number of surgeons in the UK were exposed to it was in June 1990. Over 350 surgeons attended three laparoscopic cholecystectomy symposia and – surprisingly – established senior surgeons appeared much more enthusiastic than surgeons in training. Perhaps the latter group felt excluded at the outset, as it was their more experienced colleagues who attended the symposia and subsequent courses.

Diagnostic laparoscopy is unfamiliar to most general surgeons who, until recently, found little use for it in their practice. The techniques of laparoscopic surgery, similar to those of therapeutic endoscopy and traditional laparotomy, were not usually included in general surgical training. Laparoscopic cholecystectomy very quickly became established as one of the accepted treatments for gallstones and, as it involved techniques different from those acquired during a general surgeon's training period, it was agreed that specific training was necessary and should be structured to ensure safe performance from the start of operation. It was found from the first survey that the younger surgeons in training felt that accreditation was necessary. Most of them were also concerned that the operation was being performed at that time by inexperienced consultants.

Despite the success of the early symposia in the UK, and also in the USA, it was soon realized that this was not the way to teach minimal access surgery. It whetted the appetite, but laboratory work with trainers could only teach surgeons how to use instruments and learn co-ordination. This is vital, but it is better taught in small groups and basic courses were quickly devised around the world. In the UK, the newly founded Society of Minimally Invasive General Surgeons arranged two-day laparoscopic cholecystectomy courses around the country in an attempt to standardize the training which was being offered in different ways at different hospitals. These courses included didactic lectures, training on simulators and assisting in the operating theatre (*see* Table 17.14).

PROGRAMME

0830	REGISTRATION
0850	Welcome and introduction
0900	Video of laparoscopic cholecystectomy
0920	Instruments and theatre design
0940	Anaesthetic, creation and maintenance of pneumoperitoneum and complications
1000	Lasers, principles and safety
1020	COFFEE
1040	Laser delivery systems
1100	Demonstrations and instruction on laparoscopic simulators
1230	LUNCH
1330	Laparoscopic cholecystectomy demonstration and assisting in theatre
1700	Ward round and case discussion
1930	COURSE DINNER

DAY TWO

0800	Ward round
0830	Coffee and theatre – assisting with laparoscopic cholecystectomies (Theatres 3 and 7)
1230	LUNCH
1330	Laparoscopy in the acute abdomen
1400	Training on laparoscopic simulators Theatre – assisting with laparoscopic cholecystectomies (Theatre 3)
1600	Other general surgery laparoscopic procedures
1630	Difficulties and solutions
1700	COURSE ENDS

Table 17.14: Course for laparoscopic cholecystectomy.

At about this time, guidelines were being laid down by colleges and societies (*see* Tables 17.15–17.18). The Canadian Association of General Surgeons also issued a policy on laparoscopic surgery (*see* Table 17.18).

For those without residency training or fellowship which included laparoscopic surgery, or without documented prior experience in laparoscopic surgery, the basic minimum requirements for training should be:

a. completion of approved residency training in general surgery

b. credentialling in diagnostic laparoscopy

c. training in laparoscopic general surgery by a surgeon experienced in laparoscopic surgery, or completion of a university-sponsored or academic society-recognized didactic course with clinical experience and hands-on laboratory practice

d. observation of laparoscopic surgical procedures performed by a surgeon (or surgeons) experienced in the performance of such procedures.

Table 17.15: Excerpt from the Society of American Gastrointestinal Endoscopic Surgeons' guidelines: *Granting of privileges for laparoscopic (peritoneoscopic) general surgery*.

Individuals who perform laparoscopic cholecystectomy should:

a. be trained general surgeons with current competence in performance of open cholecystectomy and in the management of the predictable complications of the operation

b. have expertise in laparoscopy acquired through previous clinical experience or through instruction

c. have completed an experience in supervised performance of laparoscopic cholecystectomy which included instruction and practice on animals

d. provide notification to their patients of the surgeon's experience with and the status of the procedure.

Table 17.16: The Society for Surgery of the Alimentary Tract's recommendations for the training and credentialling aspects of laparoscopic cholecystectomy.

For a surgeon to be granted privileges to perform laparoscopic cholecystectomy, the following requirements must be met:

1. The surgeon must be privileged to perform biliary tract operations through an accredited residency programme in general surgery.

2. The surgeon must be privileged in diagnostic laparoscopy. For those not privileged, privileging requires all of the following:

    a. tutoring by someone already privileged in laparoscopy (eg gynaecologist): in the indications, contraindications, technique, risks, complications and results of diagnostic laparoscopy

    b. participating (performing or first-assisting) in a sufficient number of procedures (minimum number: five) to become proficient in laparoscopy

    c. having the tutor certify in writing that the surgeon is competent in both the understanding and techniques of diagnostic laparoscopy.

3. The surgeon must have taken a formal course in laparoscopic cholecystectomy that includes both didactic instruction and hands-on experience on live animals.

4. The surgeon must have assisted in at least five laparoscopic cholecystectomies in humans.

5. The surgeon must be proctored by a surgeon with privileges in biliary tract surgery and/or laparoscopic cholecystectomy in at least three laparoscopic cholecystectomies. The proctor must certify in writing that the surgeon is competent to perform the procedure.

6. Provisional privileges in laparoscopic cholecystectomy may be granted by the Division Chief of General Surgery after the completion of requirement 4, but full privileges will not be recommended to the Executive Committee of the Medical Staff and the Board of Trustees until completion of requirement 5.

Table 17.17: Abington Memorial Hospital criteria for granting of clinical privileges in laparoscopic cholecystectomy (based on the guidelines of the Royal College of Surgeons of England).

1. Only general surgeons experienced with open cholecystectomy and management of its potential complications should perform laparoscopic cholecystectomy.

2. Laparoscopy should be learned through appropriate instruction.

3. The individual should have completed and experienced supervised performance in a structured course of laparoscopic cholecystectomy, or completed
   a formal general surgery residency program which includes laparoscopic
   cholecystectomy. The individual must observe and take part in the performance
   of the procedure in humans with individuals already fully experienced.

4. The training programs in laparoscopic cholecystectomy must be developed
   and located in University Centres throughout Canada and should be
   coordinated through the surgical chairmen and/or general surgical division
   chairmen. GAGS endoscopy committee would be available for resource
   purposes.

5. Training for laparoscopic cholecystectomy should be available to all interested
   general surgeons.

Table 17.18: Guidelines for laparoscopic cholecystectomy issued by the Canadian
Association of General Surgeons.

Definitions[5]

Not all words used in the American medical literature on training are
commonly used in Europe.

Certification is proof that a physician has accomplished a residency training
programme, been involved in basic didactic activities, achieved a technical
knowledge of that particular specialty and passed an examination in that
specialty. This is confirmed by a signed statement provided by the residency
programme director.

Credentials are written documentation of specific training or experience, eg
a certificate of attendance at a teaching course, symposium or even a medical
school diploma.

Competence is the minimum level of experience and skill necessary for a
physician to be able to care for patients within a specialty or to perform
certain technical procedures or operations.

Clinical privileges are the functions and procedures that the physician is
allowed to perform in the course of caring for patients in a given hospital.
Granting clinical privileges will ensure that patients receive skilful treatment
by highly qualified and competent surgeons.

Since laparoscopic surgical procedures involve techniques which have not
been familiar to most general surgeons, surgical leaders have the responsibility
of determining what constitutes adequate training for their safe performance,
and to recommend the necessary criteria. With this in mind, new basic

courses have been devised, which include theoretical as well as practical parts (*see* Tables 17.19 and 17.20). In the practical part, surgeons in training become familiar with the various instruments, optics, cameras, X-rays and energy sources. There is instruction in eye-hand co-ordination, the use of simulators or phantoms and cameras, the safe introduction of the Verres needle and trocars, and stapling and suturing techniques. As tactile input is removed and long instruments are needed, depth perception is altered. Also, the video screen picture seen is a two-dimensional representation of three-dimensional structures, and this causes further co-ordination problems. Dissection is performed on inanimate tissues. In the operating theatre, each participant on the course works in rotation as the camera operator, assistant surgeon and surgeon.

Laparoscopic cholecystectomy basic course

Historical data on laparoscopy (diagnostic and operative)

Information on equipment and instruments

Basic principles of laparoscopy

Technique of laparoscopic operations (cholecystectomy and appendicectomy)

Diagnostic procedures: cholangiography, ultrasonography

Pitfalls and complications of laparoscopic surgery

Review of results based on prospective studies and registries of laparoscopic cholecystectomy and appendicectomy

Viewing instructional videotapes

Table 17.19: Basic training in laparoscopic cholecystectomy: theory.

Part 1

Training in simulators focused on new techniques of dissection

Endoscopic suturing

Part 2

Animal experience under conditions closely resembling the actual setting

Each participant performing at least two or three different advanced endoscopic procedures and assisting

Part 3

Clinical experience (an important element of the training process) by hands-on participation in actual operating room environment

Assisting experienced surgeons in new advanced procedures (it is strongly recommended when starting advanced procedures to do so assisted by a surgeon with experience in this particular field)

Table 17.20: Basic training in laparoscopic cholecystectomy: practice.

The need to understand the equipment is of paramount importance. The technical failure of the equipment could lead to inability to perform the operation.

However, the time-honoured method of teaching surgical techniques by apprenticeship is still probably the best method. If certain video-enhanced telescopic surgical procedures are not performed in a residency programme, then a fellowship should be obtained in a service where these operations are being performed. Even with good apprenticeship training, it is felt that a structured course should be undertaken and, at a later date – probably once the basic operations have been mastered – an advanced course should also be undertaken. Our training therefore includes basic surgical training programmes with participation in a basic course of laparoscopic general surgery. We recommend the stepwise gaining of clinical experience, first as a camera person and then as an assistant, until the surgeon in training can perform operations with the assistance of an experienced surgeon, while still participating in meetings, symposia and congresses dedicated to minimal access surgery.

With respect to the granting of privileges, the European Association of Endoscopic Surgery has made firm recommendations (*see* Table 17.21). They have also introduced courses in advanced endoscopic surgery, which include animal laboratories. It is possible to gain operative skills on animals in most European countries and the USA. However, it is prohibited to use animals for this purpose in the UK. There is no doubt that these animal laboratories are useful for improving techniques, although they can never mirror the operation in humans.

An understanding of the basic surgical principles, and adequate experience of most procedures within a category, are usually sufficient to become competent in other procedures within that category. On the other hand, if the use of markedly different and potentially dangerous instrumentation such as the laser or laparoscope is required in a procedure, additional training is recommended. The quality of the surgeon's performance in laparoscopic procedures, as for all other surgical procedures, should be monitored through existing quality assurance mechanisms. Although basic courses in video-enhanced telescopic surgery are still strongly recommended, it is obvious that in a few years, when these operations have become standard procedures, basic courses will no longer be necessary. However, there is a problem in some specialties where minimal access surgery is being performed but, due to super-specialization, the commonly 'first-learned' procedures are not performed. In colorectal surgery, for example, specialist colorectal surgeons, who are not general surgeons, will not have been exposed to laparoscopic cholecystectomy. For these surgeons, structured courses are very strongly recommended. Colorectal surgeons could obtain experience by performing laparoscopic appendicectomies, although this would mean being present for emergency procedures which are not commonly performed by senior surgeons. This also means that there are fewer of these more basic operations being performed by surgeons in training. Those specialties which will be using video-enhanced telescopic surgery also may not be able to obtain

1. Formal fellowship or residency training in general surgery or other surgical specialty (urology, gynaecology, thoracic etc) is a basic requirement.

2. Accomplished surgical residency of a fellowship programme incorporating structured experience in endoscopic surgery, proven by a certificate provided by the residency programme director.

   Proficiency in laparoscopic surgical procedures, or equivalent clinical judgement, obtained in a residency fellowship programme, documented by a certificate of competence if necessary.

3. For those without prior residency fellowship training in laparoscopic surgery, or without documented prior experience, the minimum requirements for training should be:

   a. completion of approved residency training in general surgery in Europe
   b. training in endoscopic general surgery by a surgeon experienced in endoscopic surgery; or completion of a didactic course in endoscopic surgery under the auspices of a university, a recognized teaching hospital or academic society, which fulfils the recommendations of EAES and includes hands-on laboratory practice and clinical experience
   c. observation of endoscopic surgical procedures performed by a surgeon (or surgeons) experienced in the performance of such procedures is strongly recommended.

4. The applicant's training in endoscopic surgery should be confirmed in writing. Applicants should fulfil criteria as mentioned in 1. Attendance at short courses which do not provide supervised hands-on experience must not be considered as sufficient for granting equivalent competency.

Table 17.21: Training and determination of competence. European Association for Endoscopic Surgery's recommendations for granting privileges for minimal access surgery.

the experience in performing laparoscopy that most societies would recommend. Urologists performing pelvic node clearances and nephrectomies would come into this category. However, if these surgeons in training are exposed to routine and emergency video-enhanced telescopic procedures before they specialize, they will be able to carry this on into their subspecialties. There is no doubt that video-enhanced telescopic surgery will become part of the standard practice of a general surgeon. It will also be part of the training of all general surgery residents. The need for teaching courses in animal laboratories will be significantly reduced, and future courses will focus mainly on new instruments and technologies.

It may be that in a few years, computer-generated virtual reality will be incorporated into surgical training. Simulators (such as used by pilots) may be adapted for training and become less expensive in the future.[6]

References

1   Cuschieri A (1990) Minimal access surgery: the birth of a new era. *J. R. Coll. Surg. Edin.* **35**:345–7.

2   Ministry of Health (1977) *Hospital inpatient inquiry for England and Wales.* HMSO, London.

3   Royal College of Surgeons Report (1990) *Minimal access surgery: laparoscopic cholecystectomy and related gastrointestinal procedures.* Invicta, Ashford.

4   Society of American Gastrointestinal Endoscopic Surgeons (1990) *Granting of privileges for laparoscopic (peritoneoscopic) general surgery.* Society of American Gastrointestinal Surgeons, Los Angeles.

5   Dent TL (1991) Training, credentialling and granting of clinical privileges for laparoscopic general surgery. *Am. J. Surg.* **161**:399–403.

6   Noah M (1991) Endoscopy simulation. *Endosc. Rev.* **8**:8–28.

18

The Future – What Next?

HANS TROIDL

'Hopeless!' was the emphatic comment of my colleague Brendan Devlin when I told him that I was writing about the future of endoscopic surgery. John C Goligher, commissioned to write about the future of surgery, approached his task with exactly the same attitude. In his second sentence he stated that his subject was impossible and could only result in humiliation. He illustrated the point with the example of Barkeley Moynihan, *'an excellent abdominal surgeon and good speaker, like Churchill. Perhaps this latter was his failing, his weakness, as he spoke so easily he may have failed to think about his subject in depth. At a major conference in 1926 he stated that surgery had reached its limit and that there were no further important technical developments to come. But since that time we have seen the evolution of thoracic, oesophageal, cardiac, vascular and transplant surgery, as well as hip replacement and the development of hepatopancreaticobiliary surgery . . . Moynihan could not have been much further from the truth.'* Perhaps I should heed John Goligher's warning.

It is astonishing that, despite this, the concept of the 'gold standard' continues to be blindly adhered to. In 1989, when the 'bushfire' of endoscopic surgery was just flickering, the specialist biliary surgeon, McSherry, wrote a paper entitled 'Cholecystectomy – the gold standard' in the *American Journal of Surgery*. A year later, when the bushfire was already ablaze, M Trede again put the case for open cholecystectomy as the gold standard, in an article for *Chirurg:* 'Ein Plädoyer für die Cholezystektomie – Gold Standard der Gallensteintherapie'.

In 1992 I was asked to write an editorial 'Ist die laparoskopische Cholezystektomie bereits als Gold Standard bei der blanden Cholezystektomie anzuerkennen?' in which I was expected to define a new gold standard. Instead, leaning on the wisdom of great men, I concluded that 'the knowledge of the present is the error of the future'!

Notwithstanding the enthusiasm of most surgeons, the feasibility of a new technique such as endoscopic surgery does not guarantee its place in the future. Nor do the number of operations performed or the length of period over which a procedure is practised. Impressive examples of this include:

- internal mammary artery ligation as a forerunner of coronary artery bypass surgery

- gastric freezing as treatment for peptic ulcer disease

- surgery for renal ptosis

- extracranial–intracranial bypass surgery for the prophylaxis of strokes.

In the 1960s and 1970s, the surgical treatment of chronic duodenal ulcers – vagotomy in all its guises – dominated world and regional conferences, journals and symposia. Even academic chairs were awarded on the basis of this exciting surgical innovation. Two factors, however, have reduced it to almost nothing: first the disease, chronic duodenal ulcer, has decreased in incidence worldwide, and secondly a powerful drug therapy came onto the market in the mid-1970s. Will laparoscopic cholecystectomy suffer a similar fate?

However, I will accept the challenge and the risk of subsequent humiliation. My enthusiasm for the possibilities of endoscopic surgery outweighs my desire to play safe.

My hypothesis is that endoscopic surgery will change medicine, and especially surgery, in a fundamental way, as we have seen in transplant surgery. In my opinion, transplant surgery has helped surgery to develop because of three factors:

1   the changes in operative techniques, particularly those developed to cope with the special problems presented by the liver
2   the increase in the knowledge of pathophysiology, in particular the needs of organ conservation and immunology
3   the changing ethics and morals of surgery, especially concerning cost-benefit, cost-effectiveness and cost-utility.

Endoscopic surgery will change surgery in general by its use of new technology. The changes in technique and the new concepts required in instrumentation will be much greater than those seen in transplantation surgery – perhaps incomparably so. This new innovation will also radically change the aims of medicine and especially of surgery. While maintaining and even improving safety and surgical effectiveness, we are able to decrease the assault on the patient before, during and after surgical intervention. My belief is that if only a small part of endoscopic surgery should survive, the concept of patient-friendly surgery will remain!

Changes resulting from the development of new technology

The most important breakthrough in endoscopic surgery has been the transmission of a picture from inside the body, via telescopes and cameras, to the television screen.

As surgeons are now working from the television screen, the picture must be sharp and with accurate colour reproduction. In the future the image will be three-dimensional. We have to learn to overcome the problems of not being able to feel the consistency of the tissues. The rigid telescopes, mostly the same length and often too long, need an effective mechanism for cleaning the lens without removal from the body cavities. The cameras should also be small and self-focusing. Without a clear picture there can be no operation.

At present it is not clear which type of diathermy (bipolar or monopolar) is best for the different steps of the operation. It has yet to be demonstrated whether argon gas or diathermy is the better alternative.

The worst aspects at present are the instruments used for suction and irrigation, and these clearly need improving.

The importance of different types of lasers still has to be proven. Here, as with other aspects of endoscopic surgery, economic factors may bring limitations.

In the future, simulators and robotics will revolutionize medicine and especially surgery. Until now, computers – even the biggest ones – have been too slow; but endoscopic surgery will push the technology forward.

Changes in instruments

With a very few exceptions, instruments advertised in glossy catalogues by big companies are unacceptably archaic. Most of them were developed around 30 years ago, mainly by gynaecologists, from the concepts of traditional surgical instruments. The limited changes in instruments so far achieved in the development of endoscopic surgery remind me of the change from a stone axe to an iron axe in earlier times!

We should ask whether new instruments need to be developed step by step (as happened with the invention of the car by the addition of an engine to the previously horse drawn carriage) or whether we should use entirely new concepts (as occurred with the use of propellers for submarines, where sail power would have been impossible). For example, in my opinion, cutting with scissors is not the way forward.

We need to develop totally new concepts for gaining access to the body cavities and for handling and extracting tissues. The concept of trocars, developed more than 40 years ago, is to me the perversion of minimal access surgery. Nor should suturing and ligation, as practised in traditional surgery, have any part in the future of endoscopic surgery. Following in footsteps does not allow one to overtake! Multifunctional instruments should be developed instead, so that different operative steps can be performed without the need to change instruments.

Changes resulting from the development of new aims

The concept of patient-friendly surgery must lead to new and revolutionary aims. Besides the specific aims of less interference with the patients by surgical intervention, pain-free therapy, less fatigue, shorter convalescence and maintenance of body image, the real revolution is that the patient's view should dominate such definitions.

Of course low operative mortality and low complication rates will remain crucial, but aspects such as recurrence rates must also be reassessed. Nowadays, recurrence of a condition can often again be dealt with endoscopically. Ectopic pregnancy, for example, previously considered so dangerous that gynaecologists performed salpingectomy ('semi-castration'), can now be managed by repeated endoscopic surgery if a further ectopic pregnancy should occur.

Endoscopic surgery is the best example of patient-friendly surgery, and this ideal will become increasingly important in medicine in general as greater consideration is given to the patient's comfort and wishes. Anaesthesia, especially general surgical anaesthesia, has often taken little regard of the patient's viewpoint. It is hoped that endoscopic surgery will change this, and that in future the patient will also have a very important role in the choice of treatment modalities.

Where will endoscopic surgery be used?

This question concerns not only surgeons but also patients and equipment manufacturers. From my introductory comments, you can see that there is no safe answer.

Even if it is correct that 80% of gynaecological procedures previously performed transabdominally and transvaginally, can today be performed endoscopically, it does not necessarily follow that the same can be achieved in general surgery. There is a world of difference between the dangers associated with uterine surgery and those in lung surgery, for example. Nearly every week new operations are described in the journals. However, who can tell whether they will be soon forgotten or the start of something new? Again, the feasibility or acceptance of a new development is no guarantee for its future. In spite of this, I feel that endoscopic surgery will have an important future in the thorax and abdomen and in emergency situations, as has already been demonstrated in orthopaedic surgery, urology and gynaecology. Endoscopic surgery will have a place in surgery of the anterior and posterior mediastinum, the pleural cavity, the lung, the oesophagus and even the heart.

The optimal view produced by video surgery provides excellent facilities for diagnosis and treatment in the thorax. The only limitations on the feasible procedures in the thorax are the instruments currently available.

In the abdomen, there will be good indications for endoscopic surgery on the diaphragm, abdominal oesophagus, stomach, small bowel and colon. Some of these procedures are already being tested.

As far as I am concerned, the most exciting possibility lies in the future of endoscopic surgery in emergencies, both in the thorax and abdomen. The future rests with combining diagnosis and treatment. Diagnostic endoscopic procedures may compete with ultrasound and CT-scanning. This is reminiscent of the superiority of flexible endoscopy over radiology in providing both the means of diagnosis and therapy in the gastrointestinal tract.

I believe that another possibility for the future lies in the combination of mini-laparotomy with the views provided by the laparoscope.

A further hope is that endoscopic surgery may allow treatment of conditions previously considered inoperable. This is comparable to the treatment of tracheo-oesophageal fistulae by intubation and the stenting of biliary strictures following the introduction of flexible endoscopy.

Dangers

However, we must avoid taking new developments too far and using them inappropriately. We must never forget the principle of 'patient-friendly' surgery in our enthusiasm for the new procedures: each new advance must be assessed according to whether it is in the best interests of the patient. I believe that the current talk of specialist endoscopic surgeons represents a further danger.

Even in the Western world, health care places a great burden on a nation's economy. We must take care that endoscopic surgery does not become prohibitively expensive. However, a first-class service will not be available at a budget price.

History teaches us that every new treatment creates is own iatrogenic diseases – as has happened with the treatment of renal ptosis and autonomic nerve surgery for fatigue. We must be careful that endoscopic surgery does not do the same.

There is another warning — and a most important one! We must be careful not to allow endoscopic surgery to become like orthopaedic surgery and be industry driven. There is no doubt that co-operation between industrialists and surgeons is one way to evaluate endoscopic surgery. However, only surgeons and their learned societies should be involved in it. A business man should never decide on the basis of profit what qualifies as an 'idea' in surgery. It is only surgeons who will be held responsible for any mistakes made.

(Translator: M.A. Stebbing)

Index